CW00548245

THE HISTORY OF
EPILEPTIC THERAPY

THE HISTORY OF
EPILEPTIC THERAPY

An account of how medication was developed

D.F. Scott

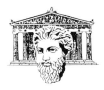

The Parthenon Publishing Group
International Publishers in Medicine, Science & Technology

Casterton Hall, Carnforth,
Lancs, LA6 2LA, UK

One Blue Hill Plaza, Pearl River,
New York 10965, USA

Published in the UK by
The Parthenon Publishing Group Limited
Casterton Hall, Carnforth,
Lancs, LA6 2LA, England

Published in the USA by
The Parthenon Publishing Group Inc.
One Blue Hill Plaza,
PO Box 1564, Pearl River,
New York 10965, USA

Copyright © 1993 Parthenon Publishing Group Ltd

British Library Cataloguing in Publication Data

Scott, Donald Fletcher
    History of Epileptic Therapy : Account of
    How Medication Was Discovered
    I. Title
    616.8

    ISBN 1-85070-391-4

Library of Congress Cataloging-in-Publication Data

Scott, Donald F.
    A history of epileptic therapy : an account of how medication was
discovered / D.F. Scott
        p.   cm.
    Includes bibliographical references and index.
    ISBN 1-85070-391-4
    1. Epilepsy—History.   2. Epilepsy—Chemotherapy—History.
3. Anticonvulsants—History.   I. Title.
    [DNLM: 1. Epilepsy—drug therapy.   2. Epilepsy—history. WL 11.1
S425h]
RC372.S345   1993
616.8'53061'09—dc20
DNLM/DLC
for Library of Congress   92-14084
                                                              CIP

First published 1993

No part of this book may be reproduced in any form without
permission from the publishers except for the quotation of brief
passages for the purposes of review

Composed by Ryburn Typesetting Ltd, Halifax
Printed and bound in Great Britain by
Butler and Tanner Ltd., Frome and London

Contents

*The book is dedicated
with love to my late wife and family
for their tolerance during the writing*

Preface

The idea of this book arose because of my increasing personal interest in the changing pattern of epilepsy, over 25 years of treating patients, mainly those who presented problems because of the chronicity of the disorder. During this time I have seen the impact of the introduction of new compounds, followed later by decline in their use and even deletion from the pharmacopoeia. Also, I have noted the changing face of epilepsy with, for example, a decrease in the incidence of status epilepticus. Perhaps more importantly, in relation to drug therapy itself, was the realization that my emphatic statements about continuing advances were not borne out in practice. I confidently wrote in the first edition of *About Epilepsy* (1965) that new drugs were being discovered and the future for the patient with a chronic disorder was bright. In fact, when preparing a revised edition of the book in 1973[1] it was clear that nothing major on the drug front had emerged in the intervening period.

Even today, although important advances are in the making, we await the arrival of the miracle cure, hence the resurgence of the surgery of epilepsy, employing the newer technologies which are now available. Because of these various ideas, it seemed worth exploring what has happened previously in terms of how therapeutic agents were discovered. This is the central theme of the book.

However, it is obviously necessary to consider the history of epilepsy to some extent, bearing in mind the comment of the essential figure in the field, Hughlings Jackson, who wrote 'we must remember that many doctrines were stated years ago in principle. They were then novel and much disputed, but are now so generally accepted that we are in danger of ceasing to think of the very early propounders of those doctrines'[2].

A full account of the early history of epilepsy is given in Owsei Temkin's *The Falling Sickness*[3] and this is recommended to the reader. The lists of references at the end of each chapter, which are comprehensive, though not exhaustive, provide sources for those who wish to delve more deeply into these, or other aspects of the subject. Fortunately it has been possible to insert some recently discovered material on historical aspects from Babylon, India and China, of particular interest because they pre-date the writings of the Hippocratic school.

In this book I have brought together material from very diverse sources, to give as coherent a narrative of the discovery of drugs as is currently possible. For those treating patients with epilepsy the third edition of *Anti-Epileptic Drugs* edited by Levy and colleagues is essential reading[4]. It shows incidentally that some compounds have appeared, only to be removed from the pharmacopoeia at a later date. Perhaps surprisingly, the full story of the discovery of phenytoin was not available until as recently as 1985, some 50 years after its discovery. Obviously, for more recent drugs the story is incomplete, but I have been aided in this connection with valuable information from many manufacturers whose help I warmly acknowledge. I have emphasized the influence in these discoveries of chance, luck, and serendipity, which I have labelled the 'casino factors', and have traced their importance in more recent advances, where there has been a move from the empirical to the rational approach. This applies equally in other fields of therapeutics, in relation to antibiotics and anticancer drugs to mention just two areas. The development of animal models, which has been essential in drug discoveries for epilepsy as well as in other parts of medicine, has also, surprisingly, been subject to the vagaries of chance and luck, and these have been discussed.

I have not been daunted in writing about newer compounds, several of which are still not available on prescription, as well as giving some account as is necessary, albeit simplified, of the bio-chemical and neurophysiological substrates of epilepsy. In the course of this book I have linked most drugs to some aspect of the management of epilepsy, so that there is mention of investigatory techniques such as electroencephalography and neuroradiology. Benzodiazepines are linked with status epilepticus, and the psycho-tropic effects of carbamazepine in those who do not have seizures, but a primary psychiatric disorder, are also discussed. For these reasons this book is not always chronological but it is hoped that the main theme, progress in antiepileptic treatment, is constantly in the forefront.

This book deals with the major current antiepileptic compounds, and to avoid a mere catalogue of drugs used, those that have been discovered and superseded, though important in their time, have received relatively scant attention here. Incidentally, I have generally used the non-proprietary name now employed, even though not the first one actually used. There is another point that must be mentioned. This concerns the date when a drug was introduced. It varies from source to source, because the date relates not just to the earliest reports but also to when the regulatory authorities gave permission for it to be available on prescription.

Having reached this point it seemed logical to attempt, using a crystal ball, to look into the future! For this I have drawn parallels with other neurological and chronic disorders in which the same type of problem in treatment is found. The vision that I perceive for the future is optimistic rather than ecstatic.

I have found the task of writing this book engrossing and I hope some of my enthusiasm will be conveyed to the reader. In terms of numbers affected, a drug for epilepsy, even though it is a chronic disorder, is by no means as important as therapeutic agents for cancer or vascular disease. Nevertheless, I hope this account will be seen as a microcosm, because it does appear that drugs in other areas have been discovered and developed in a relatively similar manner, the 'casino factors' operating elsewhere also.

This book should not only be of interest to those who care for people with epilepsy, from the medical professionals, the neurologists and psychiatrists, through to the social workers and the leaders of patient action groups, but also to the physicians in other areas and pharmacologists, as well as those who are interested in the history of medicine in general. This is a field of expanding interest, with symposia on various historical aspects and a new journal on the history of neurosciences soon to be published.

Finally, I would not have written this book without the help of so many colleagues who have offered advice and suggestions. Thanks must also go to the librarians of The Royal London Hospital for searches of relevant material, in particular Brenda Malone, to Dr John

Mumford of Merrel Dow and my publishers without whose continuing interest this task would never have been completed. I am grateful to Franz Niclaus for the translation of Hauptmann's paper on Luminal, the basis of Chapter 4, and for his attempts, sadly unsuccessful, to locate a portrait. The Medical Photography Department of the Royal Free Hospital kindly prepared the illustrations, and are warmly acknowledged. A special thanks goes to my secretary, Mrs Patricia Siddall, for typing the manuscript and indeed for her patience in re-typing many sections which proved difficult to draft. My thanks must also go to AMS for her constant help at various levels, from the conception to the completion of the task.

December 1992 *Professor D.F. Scott*

REFERENCES

1. Scott, D.F. (1973). *About Epilepsy*. (London: Duckworth)
2. Jackson, J.H. and Taylor, J. (1931/32). *Selected Writings of John Hughlings Jackson*, vol 1 and 2. (London: Hodder and Stoughton). (Reprinted 1958, New York: Basic Books)
3. Temkin, O. (1945). *The Falling Sickness*. (Baltimore: John Hopkins Press). (2nd edn., 1971)
4. Levy, R. *et al*. *Antiepileptic Drugs*. 3rd edn. (New York: Raven)

1

Introduction

There is obviously more to the management of epilepsy than using antiepileptic medication. Accurate diagnosis and the appreciation of the individual's overall social setting are just two of the other essentials in the equation. Epilepsy, just because of its multifactorial nature, can be of continuing interest, especially at the present time because of new advances in drug therapy and other possibilities such as neural grafting. Nevertheless, it is humbling to peruse the history of the condition, to see the depths of understanding of many earlier physicians in various parts of the world. In spite of the panoply of 20th century technology and pharmacology, there are still areas in which knowledge has advanced little from the views, for example, of the 1st century BC or the mid-19th century physician. This historical panorama is admirably reviewed by Temkin[1] in his book *The Falling Sickness* (see Figure 1). However, these excursions backwards in time often lead us to smile and even laugh at earlier methods of treatment, in particular at the infinite variety of substances given to aid the sufferer, as well as other therapeutic manoeuvres such as blood-letting and cauterization (Figure 2 and Table 1).

In the 19th century, the pace of advance, not only concerning views on the disorder but also on medication, gathered speed. The time between one discovery and the next decreased as the 20th century dawned. The gap between the introduction of bromides in 1857 to the start of treatment with phenobarbitone in 1912 was 55 years. It was 24 years later that the pioneer work on phenytoin was carried out, and only a matter of months elapsed before it was used in treatment. After a gap in terms of major drugs, the launches of front-runners, carbamazepine and sodium valproate, were 19 years apart (see Table 2).

1

THE FALLING SICKNESS

*A History of Epilepsy from the Greeks
to the Beginnings of Modern Neurology*

BY

OWSEI TEMKIN, M. D.

*Associate Professor of the History of Medicine
at The Johns Hopkins University*

BALTIMORE
THE JOHNS HOPKINS PRESS
1945

Figure 1 Title page of *The Falling Sickness*, by Owsei Temkin (1945)[1]; the most exhaustive historical account of epilepsy from ancient times. There is also a revised 2nd edition, published in 1971. (Reproduced with kind permission from Gibbs *et al.* (1935). EEG in petit mal. *Arch. Neurol. Psychiatry*, **34**, 1134–48)

2

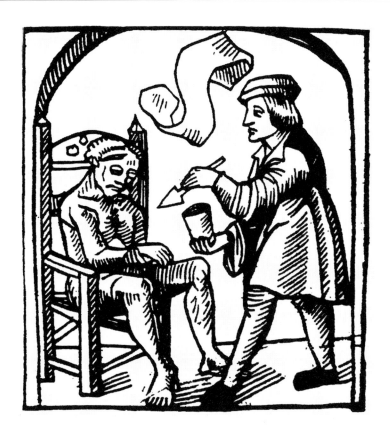

Figure 2 Treatment of King Charles II's convulsions which occurred during his terminal illness, by 'letting' one pint of blood. See Table 1 for other treatments. (Reproduced with permission from *Hospital Doctor*, 1981. Original source untraced)

At the present time there are many drugs being tested; hopefully a few will grace the pharmacy shelves in the not too distant future, and one may perhaps prove to be the miracle cure we await.

Another notable point is that of geography. One might have expected that one country would have a 'corner' in this field of chemistry, but this is not so, and many countries have played their parts (Table 3).

How antiepileptic drugs were discovered, and the route by which they reached daily use, is a fascinating story and recounting it is the main purpose of this book. It is just as important to place the drugs in their historical perspective, which we shall also do.

Table 1 Treatments administered to Charles II in his terminal illness (1685)

One pint of blood 'let from arm' (see Figure 2)
Emetic and two purgatives
Enema of antimony, sacred bitters, rock salt, mallow leaves, violets,
    beetroot, camomile flowers, fennel seed, linseed, cinnamon,
    cardamon seed and aloes
Head shaved and blistered
Sneezing powder of hellebore root
Cowslip flower powders
White wine, absinthe and anise
Extract of thistle leaves, mint rue and angelica
Plaster of Burgundy pitch and pigeon dung to the feet
Bleeding and purging continued
Extract of human skull
Mixture of Raleigh's antidote, pearl julep and ammonia

Table 2 Dates of introduction of main antiepileptic drugs currently used. Additionally, oxazolidines, for example tridione, were introduced in 1946, and succinamides, for example Miltonin, in 1953. Benzodiazepines, such as diazepam, were introduced in 1973

Year of introduction	Origin	Intervening years
1857	bromide	
		55
1912	phenobartitone	
		26
1938	diphenyl-hydantoin (phenytoin)	
		16
1954	carbamazepine	
		19
1973	valproate	
		17
1990	vigabatrin	

DRUG NAMES

Non-proprietary names have been used throughout the text. Even these may vary between countries, but this is much less so than for

4

Table 3   The geography of the main antiepileptic drugs

Potassium bromide	England
Phenobarbitone	Germany
Phenytoin	United States
Carbamazepine	Switzerland
Sodium valproate	France
Vigabatrin	France
Lamotrigine	England

labels given by the drug companies themselves, which inevitably are different from country to country, particularly in an era when promotion and sales are the handmaiden of research and development (see Chapter 12). The cost of discovery of a drug and its eventual marketing is not negligible and, though anticonvulsants provide a steady source of revenue as epilepsy is a chronic disorder, the cost of research is high, as is the testing and the presentation of the voluminous data to the regulatory authorities. This applies in all areas of medicine and leads to a delay between discovery and marketing of the order of 10 years for most compounds. Toxicity is a major consideration, and it is clear that years must unavoidably elapse from the moment of discovery to the time when the pharmacist hands a bottle of tablets to the patient. Not only that, but a number of hopeful starters in the race fall at different fences so that only a small number reach the finishing line, and of these now a miniscule proportion prove to be of major significance in therapy.

DEFINITIONS

The clinical manifestations of fits or seizures, the former more commonly used in the UK and the latter in the US, vary greatly, ranging from brief vacant spells, still called by many 'petit mal', using the French nomenclature introduced by Esquirol, to 'grand mal', a term with the same etymological background, to which the term convulsions or tonic/clonic seizures is now applied, a condition well illustrated in a 15th century medical manuscript (Figure 3).

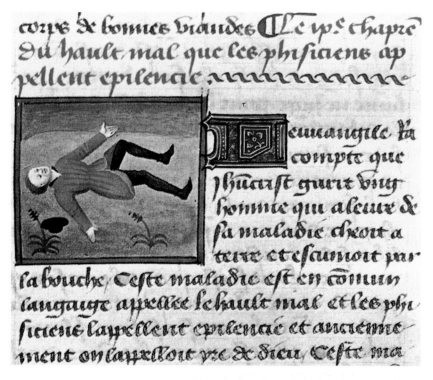

Figure 3 A miniature frontispiece from 'An Epileptic Bibliography' (in German), by N.J. Pies (1990). It is taken from *The Nature of Things* by the 15th century writer, Bartholomew, the Englishman, printed with the Latin title *De Proprietatibus Rerum* in Lyam, 1482. A copy was recently listed in a bookseller's catalogue priced at £1950. (Reproduced with kind permission of Robert Pfützner Verlag, München)

Between these extremes are a great variety of attacks resulting from focal, but spreading discharge from the cortex. Fits arising in the temporal lobe may have a similar brevity to petit mal, whilst others are much longer with a wide range of psychological and motor manifestations. Some are fragments of ordinary behaviour seen in repetitive and disorganized fashion, known as automatisms. These may be associated with memory aberrations and distortions of time sense, to give just two examples of the wide variety of psychological accompaniments of seizures. Because of the diverse nature of non-convulsive anomalies seen, it has been suggested that anti-seizure medication or antiepileptic drugs would be more appropriate terms than 'anticonvulsants', though the latter is still widely used. In this book the term antiepileptic will be employed throughout.

As to terminology in general, I have sometimes used the word 'fit'. The abrupt Anglo-Saxon nature is typical of our ancestors, who gave us short decisive words. However, these are not favoured by all; indeed even in a permissive era they are still regarded as improper. The term 'seizure' which is used interchangeably has a more generally accepted currency. A valuable word in this context is attack because it can be applied, as in this book, to episodes which may or may not be of an epileptic nature. I have also used it as a blanket term when describing manifestations of temporal lobe epilepsy, bearing in mind, as mentioned above, the variable and protean nature of the behavioural phenomena encountered when the cortical discharge arises in that location. Other terms such as psychomotor seizures may be used as a variant, although this is now 'old-fashioned' and strictly we should adhere to the International Classification as described by Gastaut[2,3]. Reference to this is essential in defining our aims, particularly in clinical trials of antiepileptic drugs (see Laidlaw and Richens[4], for discussion on classification, including recent variants). The equivalent of 'petit mal' in the International Classification is 'absence seizures'; temporal lobe attacks are simple or complex partial seizures, and convulsions, tonic/clonic fits.

Clinical trials have now advanced greatly in design and statistical analysis since the action and assessment of medication was reviewed by Coatsworth[5]. Detailed classification enables us to have treatment delineated on a more rational basis (see particularly Chapters 11 and 12). However, this rushes ahead of where we have reached so far and we must return to more fundamental matters.

HOW ARE ANTICONVULSANTS DISCOVERED?

When we attempt to clarify the nature of the discovery of antiepileptic or indeed any other medication, we enter an area more akin to the casino than the chemistry laboratory. It is for this reason that the subtitle of this book could be 'chance, luck and serendipity in the discovery of antiepileptic drugs'. This is only one aspect because compounds may be synthesized years before they are found to be useful in treatment, and time also elapses before they appear on the clinical scene, because of the need for assessing their efficacy and toxicity, and for submission to the regulatory authorities (Chapter 12).

There are indeed many reasons for this time lag, not least the necessity of providing an appropriate means of testing the drug before it is administered even to normal human volunteers. Here animal models are essential. At the present time, and rightly so, there is discussion about the use and, in some instances, the abuse of animals in experimentation (Chapter 12). However, the development of the treatment of epilepsy is one area in which discovery of medication would have been impossible without animal work. Finding appropriate models requires an understanding both of the basis of the chemical substrate of the brain and also how it may be deranged in seizure disorders. There are, as we shall see, species differences and even differences within species (see Chapter 10), which affect the choice of an appropriate model. Indeed it can be influenced almost as much by chance and luck as by an intellectual grasp of the problem.

Then which compounds should be chosen from the rows and rows of bottles on the shelves of the synthetic chemist is another matter. Also swayed by many factors, the answer must be to test them all and, indeed, re-test them in the light of changes in knowledge and methods.

Just one example of how luck must be on the side of the experimenter was the discovery of the baboon which responded to flashing lights. It was only one species from a certain area with a particular inheritance which showed this propensity (see Chapter 10). This was the appropriate model for the assessment of such dissimilar drugs as sodium valproate, diazepam and phenobarbitone.

THE 'CASINO FACTOR'

There are three elements to what I have called the 'casino factor'[6]. The first, chance, plays a part in many discoveries, not least with antiepileptics; perhaps a casual glance at a journal displayed in the library or a passing remark at a meeting may start a whole new train of thought in the experimenter's mind. Here is a crucial example in the history of epilepsy (Chapter 3). Sir Charles Locock, Queen Victoria's obstetrician, read that bromide had a beneficial effect in curbing sexual desires in a German physician. How did this lead to the use of the compound in epilepsy? The historical background, as always, is important; as Koestler observes 'there must be a ripeness of time'[7]. In this context it related to the belief that sexual activity was causative for seizures. Masturbation was a culprit[8], hence the suggestion about bromide. It would suppress this activity and control fits. Also at this time, the mid-19th century, there was an increasing search for 'specifics' for epilepsy and the era of blood-letting and purging and other such treatments was almost at an end. Elemental compounds such as zinc were regarded as possible specifics for the treatment of seizures, as was iron. These two and other elements were to stimulate the use of potassium bromide which proved to be a valuable, if toxic, drug for 50 years, as the physician waited, not knowing that barbituric acid first synthesized in 1864 was already on the organic chemists' shelves, and Luminal (phenobarbitone) would soon arrive to revolutionize the treatment even further.

Chance, derived via old French from the Latin *cadare*, to fall, is an unexpected happening without a definite cause. It may play for us or against us, whilst the second factor, luck, is different. It is from the low German word *Glück*, prosperity. This is always positive and implies good fortune, but *still* in the context of what has gone before in terms of other discoveries. Dr Tracy J. Putnam was searching for a new non-sedative drug which had anticonvulsant properties. He had a list of 19 possibles which were sent to the Parke Davis company. How he made contact with Parke Davis and the development of the animal model for testing is all part of the fascinating story (see Chapter 6), but at this point suffice it to say that the first compound on the list for testing was diphenyl-hydantoin, phenytoin.

Luck seems a trivial word when the total background is considered, but even though a new discovery rarely occurs *in vacuo*, yet we must not deny its importance. As the French writer Jean Cocteau cynically exclaimed, 'we must believe in luck. For how else can we explain the success of those we don't like'.

Serendipity is the last of the trio, an interesting word coined by Sir Horace Walpole, the writer, in 1754. It is derived from the former word for Sri Lanka (also called Ceylon in the interim) used in the title of the fairy tale called 'The Three Princes of Serendip'. They were 'always making discoveries by accident and sagacity, of things they were not in quest of'. As with so many definitions, this includes a word which itself requires that we turn to yet another page in the dictionary and so on!

'Sagacity' is in fact the key here because it implies that the people to whom serendipitous discoveries occur have to be keen in thought and perception to make use of what they find. The word serendipitous has been applied to the discovery of sodium valproate (see Chapter 10). Several compounds being screened for antiepileptic activity all showed positive effects. It was the solvent valproic acid that was the active substance, so in this way began one of the most important recent chapters in the field of the treatment of epilepsy using sodium valproate.

A HISTORICAL PERSPECTIVE

We must now return to the start of our trail, the years before Christ when much was written about epilepsy. Hippocrates is seen as an important figure (see Chapter 2). The name conjures up the idea of an impressive Greek figure. In fact the writings attributed to Hippocrates are not the work of one man, but of a school, rather in the way that the Renaissance artist collected around him students who imitated their master's work and provided an attribution, such as 'School of Titian', thus causing headaches for art historians and rapacious 20th century art auctioneers, as well as the wealthy collectors!

Whoever wrote the Hippocratic corpus obviously had a wide experience of epilepsy. As Lennox pointed out, more is devoted to epilepsy in the Hippocratic writings than in the modern textbook of medicine[9]. Clearly the importance of the subject relates not only to the number of patients who suffer, but also to the chronicity. Indeed, these patients represent perhaps a third of all those who attend the neurological outpatient department.

In the next chapter, apart from the Hippocratic corpus, we shall allude to a recently translated Babylonian text and to writings from the Far East in about the same era, continuing through the relatively barren historical route to the mid-19th century when the antiepileptic saga begins in earnest. Successive chapters will deal with the discovery of individual antiepileptic compounds, bringing us to the present time, dealing with important issues in the context of each new medication and finally predicting possible future advances (Figure 4).

Other aspects of management in relation to how they affect the whole patient will be broached, including investigation by electro-

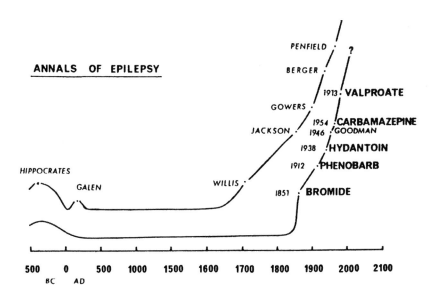

Figure 4 A graph showing the marked change in management of epilepsy over the centuries. Note the pace of increase in the discovery of antiepileptic agents on the right, and innovations on the left. (From Melville[10], with kind permission of author and publisher, modified from Lennox[9])

encephalography and neuroradiology. These advances are sometimes ahead, and sometimes lagging behind, the biochemical and pharmacological approaches. Surgery too requires mention. It flourished only to be overtaken as a result of the efforts of biochemists, but now, in the advanced technological era in which we are currently working, it is very much 'alive and well'.

Finally, we are not allowed to forget that this is an era of rapid expansion in medical treatment and specifically in neurology and psychiatry (see Chapter 12). Molecular genetics and, later, genetic engineering seem to have limitless possibilities. Consider another and not unrelated area, namely the feasibility of transplants – neural grafts – applied to neurological disorder. Parkinsonism is the first candidate in this particular area, but there are many others where enzyme deficiency in the brain is the underlying feature. Alzheimer's disease is producing a spate of activity in terms of pharmacological approaches at the present time. Here too transplants of biochemically active cells seem a strong possibility in the not too distant future.

What about epilepsy? A cluster of cells, from cadaver or test tube, capable of producing gamma-aminobutyric acid (GABA) implanted into, say, the frontal lobe may seem far fetched, but it may have already taken place by the end of the decade. Those working on transplants need chance on their side. They require all the luck in the world and must have a keen perception not to be startled by the hallucination of The Three Princes of Serendip when their ancient Ceylonese barque floats into view!

To conclude, it must be emphasized at this point that much has been written about the history of epilepsy in general, whilst the antiepileptic drugs themselves have received relatively scant attention[10], so here we will concentrate on medication *per se*. Clearly, this must be set in an historical perspective, and in the next chapter concepts of management put forward in the first millenium BC and before will be discussed, as well as the story in the Roman era and mediaeval times. This brings us (see Chapter 3) to the beginning of the true era of medical treatment in the mid-1880s.

REFERENCES

1. Temkin, O. (1945). *The Falling Sickness*. (Baltimore: Johns Hopkins Press). (2nd edn., 1971)
2. Gastaut, H. (1969). Clinical and electroencephalographical classification of epileptic seizures. International league against epilepsy. *Epilepsia*, **10** (Suppl.), S2
3. Gastaut, H. (1969). Classification of the epilepsies. *Epilepsia*, **10** (Suppl.), S14
4. Laidlaw, J. and Richens, A. (1982). Introduction. *Textbook of Epilepsy*. (Edinburgh: Churchill)
5. Coatsworth, J.J. (1971). Studies on the clinical efficacy of marketed anti-epileptic drugs. NINDS Monograph, **12**. (Bethesda, Maryland: US Dept. Health, Education and Welfare)
6. Spanier, D. (1988). *Easy Money Inside the Gambler's Mind*. (London: Abacus, Sphere Books)
7. Koestler, A. (1964). *Act of Creation*. (London: Huchinson)
8. Hare, E.H. (1962). Masturbatory insanity. *J. Ment. Sci.*, **108**, 1
9. Lennox, W.G. (1960). *Epilepsy and Convulsive Disorders*. (Boston: Little Brown)
10. Melville, I.D. (1982). The medical treatment of epilepsy: a historical review. In Rose, C.T. and Bynum, W.F. (eds.) *Historical Aspects of the Neurosciences*. (New York: Raven)

2

The history of epilepsy to AD 1850

This book is mainly about the discovery of anti-convulsant drugs. However, it is necessary to put the subject in an historical context, hence this chapter considers not only the causes of epilepsy, but also its treatment and prognosis before specific drugs were discovered.

Almost all accounts start with Hippocrates, conjuring up an image, perhaps a marble statue, of a learned physician who masterminded a collection of books covering many aspects of medicine. This is at variance with the historical facts. It is true that Hippocrates (Figure 1) actually existed, being born on the Greek island of Kos in 460 BC. The island was one of the famous centres for medicine but by no means the only one in Greece or indeed in the ancient world. The Babylonians made a contribution to the understanding of epilepsy. Tablets exhibited in the British Museum for many years have recently been translated and reveal, as we shall see later, a wonderful range of descriptions of epileptic phenomena[2]. From Egypt there is documentary evidence, the Edwin–Scott papyrus, dated 1600 BC which includes case histories, suggesting that they were ahead of their Greek counterparts. Indeed, the Greeks probably had access to, and made use of, Egyptian records.

Though these remains from the Middle East show an impressive grasp of medicine, the Hippocratic corpus, the term used by scholars for these works from Kos, remain the earliest organized body of medical knowledge. Almost certainly, as Lloyd suggests[3], this represents a new phenomenon in the ancient world.

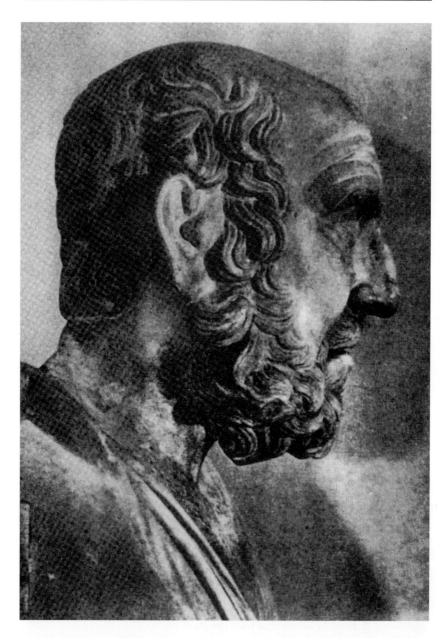

Figure 1 Bust of Hippocrates (460–377 BC), from the Uffizi Gallery, Florence. (Reproduced, with kind permission of the Clarendon Press, from *A Short History of Medicine* by Singer and Underwood[1])

14

THE HIPPOCRATIC CONTRIBUTION

The Hippocratic works not only deal with diagnosis but also prognosis. This was regarded as an important aspect of medical work since the doctors of the time were often under threat, having no organized teaching system or governmental backing of the type so valuable currently for the medical profession and the development of health care in general. The ability of a physician to make an accurate prognosis could maintain his status. Prognosis therefore receives considerable attention in the Hippocratic corpus. The basis of medicine in terms of anatomy, physiology and pathology was rudimentary, with little interest in dissection and other methods which are clearly essential for accurate diagnosis. Management of disease was limited to a regimen of prevention by protection from the climatic elements, dietary advice and programmes of rest and exercise.

Historical scholars of this period report that the Hippocratic works were from several, perhaps many, different authors. This is the view of Lloyd[3] and it is the translations of the Hippocratic works by Chadwick and Mann that are quoted throughout this chapter. Some contributors to the works lived well before the first millenium BC when Hippocrates was alive, and the books themselves had different purposes and audiences. Some are practical, others more theoretical. They range from formal lectures intended not just for doctors, but also for intelligent laymen, others are notebooks such as the 'Aphorisms' in which epilepsy is mentioned.

The first entry, although well-known, merits repetition, because it includes the responsibilities of the physician, as well as his dedication to the healing arts.

'Life is short, science is long; opportunity is elusive, experiment is dangerous, judgement is difficult. It is not enough for the physician to do what is necessary, but the patient and the attendants must do their part as well and circumstances must be favourable.'

Another aphorism concerns the treatment of epilepsy and the view put forward is that heat and cold and climatic conditions in general are important. These views persisted well into mediaeval times.

15

'The chief factor in the cure of epilepsy in the young is change, especially that due to growing up, but seasonal change of climate, or change of place or mode of life, are also important.'

There are many other references to epilepsy and convulsions but it is the book of the 'sacred disease' which is of most interest. It begins:

'I do not believe that the 'sacred disease' is any more divine or sacred than any other disease, but, on the contrary, has specific characteristics and a definite cause. Nevertheless, because it is completely different from other diseases, it has been regarded as a divine visitation for those who, being only human, view it with ignorance and astonishment. This theory of divine origin, though supported by the difficulty of understanding the malady, is weakened by the simplicity of the cure, consisting merely of ritual purification and incantation. If remarkable features in a malady were evidence of divine visitation, then there would be many 'sacred diseases' as I shall show.'

This paragraph implies that other views were current, and clearly previous medical opinion had suggested that there was indeed something special, perhaps divine, about epilepsy. Individuals had fits and the cause was in dispute. As diagnosis was a problem, so was treatment. The reason why we refer to Hippocratic books is not least because the Greeks had an understanding of what had gone before, and they clearly wrote down their own beliefs, within the historical context.

So what were the already established notions? There appears to have been quite a definite idea that epilepsy was a disorder which had a malignant cause. It arose as a result of spirits, demons and witches, against which treatment as such was of little avail. Indeed, this particular thread runs through the whole of the history of epilepsy until the more modern neurological approaches emerge in the middle, and particularly towards the end, of the 19th century.

It is intriguing that the writings of the Hippocratic school were subsequently amended, so even physicians working two centuries later were uncertain as to which should be attributed to Hippocrates and his fellow physicians and which to later alterations and additions. Until the arrival of the printing press, manuscripts, whether of a medical or religious nature, were hand-copied and this led to constant modifications, not necessarily with benefit to the original authors.

The name of Hippocrates nevertheless represents an important milestone in the story of epilepsy. These writings are still highly regarded even though the authorship is not definite, rather in the way that unattributed editorials in newspapers or medical journals are often read avidly even though their authorship is uncertain.

The Hippocratic school attacked the concept that epilepsy was related to possession by spirits, which in ancient times were thought of as benign or malignant. The idea that this was the cause of epilepsy was totally repudiated. The assertion that epilepsy was a sacred disease led the physician, according to the Greek writers, into other dangers. It enabled him to screen himself from failure to give an effective therapy, because of ignorance concerning causation. As a result, a wide range of treatments were suggested including purifications, incantations and abstinence from baths and certain foods. Perhaps more strangely, the patients were forbidden to wear black because it was a sign of death, or to use woollen blankets made from goat fleeces. If these treatments, which at least could do no harm, were ineffective, then the gods could be blamed and the physicians exonerated.

The physiological basis of epilepsy

The other significant contribution to the understanding of epilepsy in the Hippocratic writings is the affirmation concerning the physiological basis of the disorder:

'The brain is the seat of this disease as it is of other very violent disease.'

What then follows is an interesting account of the brain.

'The human brain, as in the case of all other animals, is double; a thin membrane runs down the middle and divides it. This is the reason why headache is not always located in the same site but may be on either side, or sometimes affects the whole head.'

The anatomy of the cardiovascular system is then described and its links to the brain.

'A large vessel ... disappears close to the ear and then divides; a larger part finishes in the brain ...'.

It is then clearly affirmed:

'It is through the blood vessels that we respire ... air cannot remain still but must move; if it remains still and is left behind in some part of the body then that part is powerless.'

Other physiological matters

The discourse continues with a discussion of other physiological matters, in particular bile and phlegm; their presumed importance in the causation of disease, including epilepsy, persisted in various forms for many centuries. Though the physiological basis was not fully understood, the clinical phenomena were clearly described.

'Should these routes for the passage of phlegm from the brain be blocked, the discharge enters the blood vessels which I have described. This causes loss of voice, choking, foaming at the mouth, clenching of the teeth and convulsive movements of the hands; the eyes are fixed, the patient becomes unconscious and in some cases passes a stool'.

As the discussion develops it becomes clear that lack of air in the brain was regarded as responsible for attacks, indeed quite a convincing account is given of what we now fully recognize as anoxic convulsions. Age as an important factor is also noted, as well as the difference between children and adults.

'Adults neither die from an attack of this disease nor does it leave them with any palsy.'

Auras and triggers

In both Hippocratic writings and in those from Babylon (see below) there was a clear knowledge of premonitory features of the attack. With careful reading it is possible to separate what would now be regarded as the prodrome, sometimes hours, from the brief aura, as we now regard it, merely seconds in duration and, electrically at least, the beginning of an attack.

In the Hippocratic text, precipitation is linked to certain situations. Definite advice is given here, so that the patients who suffer from 'premonitory indication of an attack' are told to avoid company, if possible to return home, or if not, to find somewhere to be on their own. From this directive it is clear that not only is preventing an attack important, but also the adverse social significance of the disorder is underlined. Mere embarrassment was only part. There was a great concern also because other people were fearful of the demon or other malignant forces, who they saw as causing the seizure.

Origin of emotions

The Hippocratic physicians were not blinkered in their view of the importance of the brain. This is well expressed in the following paragraph:

> 'It ought to be generally known that the source of our pleasure, merriment, laughter and amusement, as of our grief, pain, anxiety and tears is none other than the brain. It is specially the organ which enables us to think, see and hear and to distinguish the ugly and the beautiful, the bad and the good, pleasant and unpleasant. Sometimes we judge according to convention; at other times according to the perceptions of expediency. It is the brain too which is the seat of madness and delirium, of the fears and frights which assail us, often by night, but sometimes even by day.'

In the following quotation we see the preoccupation with temperature and humidity, these being regarded as important factors. This concern was present in many of the writings from ancient times, persisting almost until the first effective anticonvulsant drug, bromide, was discovered in the 1850s.

> 'All such things result from an unhealthy condition of the brain; it may be warmer than it should be, or it might be colder, or moister or drier, or in any other abnormal state. Moistness is the cause of madness, for when the brain is abnormally moist, it is necessarily agitated and this agitation prevents sight or hearing being steady. Because of this, varying visual and acoustic sensations are produced, while the tongue can only describe things as they appear and sound. So long as the brain is still, a man is in his right mind.'

Treatment

The Greeks, in common with other ancient medical writers, recommended a combination of dietary restrictions as well as programmes
of exercise and rest for the treatment of epilepsy. These were the
mainstay of management of seizures as well as of many other
disorders. Serious consideration was given to temperature and other
climatic factors, and to whether a change of place and mode of life
might prove helpful. Certainly contemporary studies in the twentieth
century on changes in life events have shown that this concern is not
unimportant in many serious medical disorders, even when specific
therapy is available. While in the Hippocratic corpus it is stated that
drugs can be used, there is little detailed information. This lack of
detail on therapy was interestingly criticized by later physicians who
wished to follow the methods suggested. The importance of diet in
diverse conditions was well appreciated by the ancients, and must not
be totally ignored as a form of treatment for a variety of disorders
even now. Indeed in the mid-twentieth century the ketogenic diet was
highly regarded as a method of treatment for petit mal, especially (see
Chapter 5), although it is now eclipsed again by effective medicaments.

Greek physicians did not despise the religious aspects of epilepsy,
even though firmly believing that they were not causative. In fact they
positively invoked spiritual help. Sufferers were told to sleep in the
temples of Ascelapius, the god of medicine, and healing of their
disorders and cure of epilepsy could occur. Though the Hippocratic
corpus lacks specificity in aspects of treatment, at least one particular
case of epilepsy is noted. Convulsions occurred in one man after he
anointed himself in a bath before the fire during the winter. He was
cured by complete abstinence from food or drink, though for how
long is not noted.

The book ends strongly as follows:

'In this disease as in all others, it should be your aim not to make
the disease worse, but to wear it down by applying the remedies
most hostile in the disease and those to which it is unaccus-
tomed. A malady flourishes and grows in its accustomed
circumstances but it is blunted and declines when attacked by a
hostile substance. A man with the knowledge of how to produce
by means of regimen, dryness and moisture, cold and heat in the

human body, could cure this disease too provided that he could distinguish the right moment for the application of the remedies. He would not need to resort to purifications and magic spells.'

The Hippocratic Oath

In the Hippocratic writings there is consideration of ethical behaviour. Most notable of course is the Hippocratic Oath. However, there is also discussion of fees, both for those engaged in training practitioners as well as for services to patients. This was not new. Fees had been set out in the Hammurabi code a century earlier. The payments for various operations depended on the patients' social class. For slaves they were less than for those who were free men. Perhaps we forget that Hippocrates himself became famous in his own day and as a doctor he was able to establish himself as a teacher and obtain commensurate fees.

It was partly for this reason that the doctors of the time were regarded as moneymakers, indeed many became rich. They attempted to establish themselves as practitioners to cure illness, and then they had the right to obtain fees. Their position was strengthened as a result, so that they could offer training to others and be paid for their services. Nevertheless in the Hippocratic writings there is an indication that, though it is usual to charge patients for treatment, it can be given free. Further discussion on what the patients would be charged should come late rather than early in the consultation, for fear of increasing anxiety. Many of the doctors of that time were itinerant, which obviously helped to spread their fame abroad, assuming that they were successful in treatment, as well as giving accurate predictions concerning the outcome of the patient's illness. Others, however, were employed by particular cities and were given fees for being responsible for the health of the inhabitants.

BABYLONIAN MEDICINE

Running in parallel with Greek medicine was that in Middle Eastern civilizations including Babylon[2]. A Babylonian stone tablet which has been in the British Museum for many years has recently been translated, and almost certainly represents the earliest recorded account of epilepsy. It reveals interesting insights into the physicians' view of epilepsy and its clinical ramifications. They are equally as advanced as those of the contemporary Greek practitioners, or possibly more so. The tablet (Figures 2 and 3) comes from a series of 40 tablets originally part of a Babylonian textbook of diagnostic medicine known as Sakkiku, and each tablet is the equivalent of a chapter in a modern textbook. It is dated approximately to around 500 BC but is a copy from the original compiled between the years 1067 and 1046 BC.

The translation reveals that the Babylonians, like their Greek counterparts, were concerned that the manifestations of epilepsy were the work of demons and ghosts. The concept of possession by these malignant spirits was important and it is of interest that the word 'to possess' was also the word 'to seize'.

Such possession, according to Wilson, Kinnier and Reynolds[2] in the case of the major seizure and the rationale behind it, is relatively easy to understand. The attack began with the aura, continued through to the fall itself, and reached a climax at the end of the tonic stage, the ensuing clonic stage being already a release and the beginning of the demon's departure from the body. At the end of this period the demon departs completely.

Another topic, 'ghosts', receives attention in the Babylonian text. Ghosts roam at night and phrases like 'seized by ghost' and 'hand of the ghost' were, according to Wilson, Kinnier and Reynolds[2], terms for nocturnal seizures. A distinction is made by the writer from the seizures that occur in the daytime. This is still a matter of great interest, and indeed Janz, in 1962, used this as a basis for classification of attacks[4]. There is a clear recognition of other features of the attacks. Fleeting absences, deviation of the head and eyes, simple and complex automatisms, and many other such individual and distinctive 'signs' of the seizure disorder are duly noted and written down. Additionally, the number of seizures or possessions that might afflict the epileptic person over a period of time is recorded, and whether there is a discernible and relevant pattern to the attacks.

Features of temporal lobe epilepsy are reported; epigastric auras and auditory hallucinations with buzzing, hissing, whistling and ringing were recognized then as they are today. Their significance was emphasized in the second half of the 19th century by Hughlings Jackson, being amplified later by the use of the electroencephalograph (see Chapter 5).

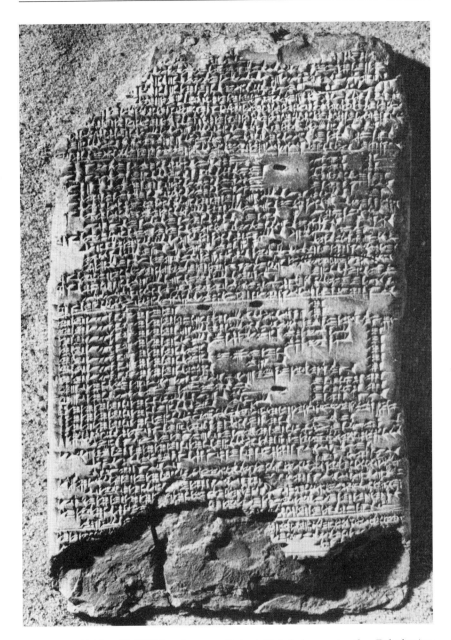

Figure 2 Tablet BM47733, obverse. This tablet belongs to the Babylonian Collection of the British Museum, and is dated to the first millennium BC[2]. (Reproduced by courtesy of the Trustees, copyright British Museum, London)

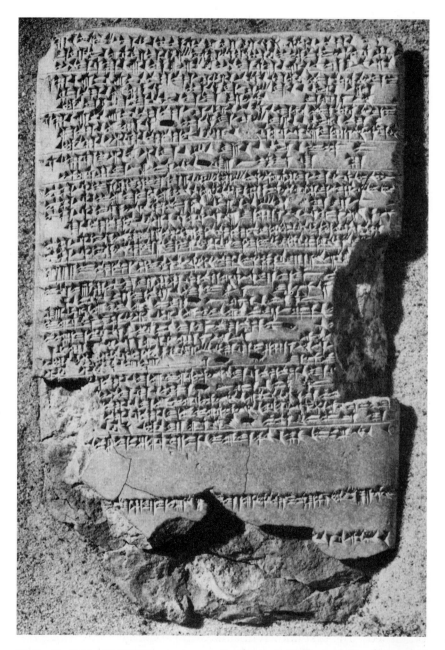

Figure 3 Tablet BM47733, reverse, see also Figure 2. (Reproduced by courtesy of the Trustees, copyright British Museum, London)

The question of serial seizures and status epilepticus, a serious condition in which one seizure follows rapidly on from another, is also mentioned. Curiously the number of attacks was thought to be important in relation to what is now called status epilepticus; seven or eight appear to be regarded as of a particularly life-threatening nature. As to the treatment, there is evidence that almost everything was tried to alleviate the disorder. Not surprisingly, in view of beliefs about causation, exorcism was used in addition to a variety of medicines, ointments, amulets and enemas.

EPILEPSY IN ANCIENT INDIAN MEDICINE

Surprisingly, it has also recently come to light that around 1500–800 BC the literature of Indian medicine dealt with neurology. Atreya, the father of Indian medical practice, defined epilepsy as a 'paroxysmal loss of consciousness', and indicated that he believed it to be a disturbance of mind, rather than due to demons and spirits. This was about 500 years before Hippocrates[5]. It is even possible that Hippocrates was aware of such views, as it is known that a contemporary of his, the physician Ctesias of Cailos, visited India. He wrote a treatise on Indian medicine. Treatment was to correct uncleanliness, which was regarded as a major aspect of the disorder; thus purges, enemas and 'vomitation' were suggested as a first step. A great variety of agents were recommended, for example, tree bark of different types cooked in clarified butter, with sour milk curds as the next line of therapy. Less savoury were various animal parts, as well as excrement, though their use indeed persisted to mediaeval times in many countries. Interestingly, protection of the patient from water, trees and mountains, was stressed repeatedly by Atreya. Resistance to treatment and the chronic nature of the disorder was well known in these ancient times.

THE ANCIENT CHINESE VIEW OF EPILEPSY

An account of Chinese medicine in ancient times has recently been published[6]. The first known document on epilepsy appeared in 'The Yellow Emperor's Classic of Internal Medicine', – 'Huang De Nei Ching', which, interestingly, like the Hippocratic corpus, was written

25

not by one but by a group of physicians around 1770–221 BC. The description of fits relates to generalized seizures without any mention of petit mal or temporal lobe attacks, that is, simple or complex partial seizures. There seems to have been difficulty in distinguishing between epilepsy and some forms of mental disorder such as psychosis and mania. Nevertheless, the description of a convulsive attack is very vivid:

> 'In the beginning of an epileptic attack the patient suddenly becomes moody, notes a heavy sensation and pain in the head, stares with eyes widely open and turning red. The patient then feels agitated. Then the epileptic attack takes off and the patient cries out and gasps ... Sometimes the attack starts out with stiffening, then the patient develops back pain (spasm?) ...'

There is also a much later description of status epilepticus in the Chinese literature, from Shen Jin Ao in AD 1776.

Classification was complex and colourful. The different types of attack were labelled after the epileptic cry made by the patient, according to which animal made a similar sound, be it goat, horse, pig, cow, chicken or dog.

The philosophy of treatment was based on a combination of specific proportions of Yang, sun energy, and Ying force; health resulted from condensation of cosmic energy.

In practice today Chinese medicine uses a traditional variety of herbs and acupuncture. The latter may include burying a piece of goat intestine into the acupuncture points. This is perhaps more reminiscent of mediaeval than modern Western medicine, yet the same physician, Yang Meng Lang, in 1983[7] also summarizes in a Chinese traditional medical textbook important points which should be considered when treating patients with epilepsy. They should be seen as frequently as possible; a description of the attack should be given by an observer; the physician may change the treatment if attacks recur, and finally questions as to precipitating factors and circumstances under which the epileptic attacks occur should be explored.

BIBLICAL CONTRIBUTIONS

There are two mentions in the New Testament of epilepsy. The first is St. Matthew's Gospel, chapter 17, verses 15–17.

'Lord have mercy on my son, for he is lunatick and sore vexed, for oftimes he falleth into the fire and oft into the water.'
'And I brought him to thy disciples and they could not cure him.'
'Then Jesus answered and said, O faithless and perverse generation, how long shall I be with you? bring him hither to me.'
'And Jesus rebuked the Devil and he departed out of him: and the child was cured from that very hour.'

This section has a number of points of interest. First of all the father regards his son as a 'lunatic', a view that persisted and indeed persists to the present day, even in the developed world. The passage indicates that the son falls into fire and water, reminding us that such dangers then as now are a serious matter. They are important to the patient and perhaps too rarely discussed by doctors, in spite of the fact that they are clearly the cause of great anxiety also to parents, relatives and friends. Indeed previous injuries are one feature indicating a poor long-term prognosis.

The next biblical reference is from St. Luke's Gospel, chapter 8, verses 38–42. Luke was reputedly a physician which may explain the discrepancies between this and the previous account.

'And behold, a man of the company cried out, saying Master I beseech thee, look upon my son: for he is mine only child.'
'And lo, the spirit taketh him and he suddenly cried out; and it reacheth him and he foamed again and bruising him hardly departeth from him.'
'And I besought thy disciples to cast him out; and they could not.'
'And Jesus answering said, O faithless and perverse generation, how long shall I be with you, and suffer you? Bring thy son hither.'
'And as he was yet coming, the devil threw him down, and tare him. And Jesus rebuked the unclean spirit, and healed the child, and delivered him again to his father.'

There is here a more detailed description of the seizure with the initial cry, but as in St. Matthew's text, there is indication of danger and possible injury. Of interest in this account is the indication of foam. In many of the early writings about epilepsy, foaming at the mouth is always emphasized, indeed still is by parents and relatives.

This was taken to extremes by regarding it as a source of infection to those who became contaminated with the foam. The result was the bracketing of epileptic sufferers with lepers, where infection was of importance, but of course not by instant contact. This erroneous view of epilepsy persisted until quite recently, and made isolation from the community in colonies seem rational, more as a 'public health measure' than an approach to care of the sufferer.

ROMAN MEDICAL WRITERS

The Roman period was noted for writers who commented on or amended earlier texts. Pliny discoursed on a wide range of subjects including medical matters but he was not particularly careful as to accuracy of quotations included with his own observations. Galen, who lived at about the same time, some 500 years after Hippocrates, was not only a voluminous writer on philosophical but also on medical subjects; these included 15 commentaries on the Hippocratic corpus. He was a careful dissector of animals and was the first to notice the pulse. However, much of his work on physiology was at a rather theoretical level. Nevertheless, he gathered together all the then current medical knowledge and became the source book for subsequent writers, even until the modern history of epilepsy and its treatments began. Indeed, Locock[8], the discoverer of the antiepileptic action of bromides, in his review of treatment talks of 'Galenics' as possible cures for the disorder.

Galen and the causes of epilepsy

Galen had definite views on certain aspects of physiology, such as the circulation of the blood (Figure 4), as well as the causation of seizures. Epilepsy according to him was divided into three groups. The first, interestingly, was labelled 'idiopathic', a term which is now frowned upon by experts but is still used widely. The seizures were caused by disturbance of humours of the brain brought on by cold. The second group was 'sympathetic'. This is worthy of note as it showed that Galen appreciated that epilepsy, though primarily a condition of the brain, could be brought on by disturbance of the body resulting in

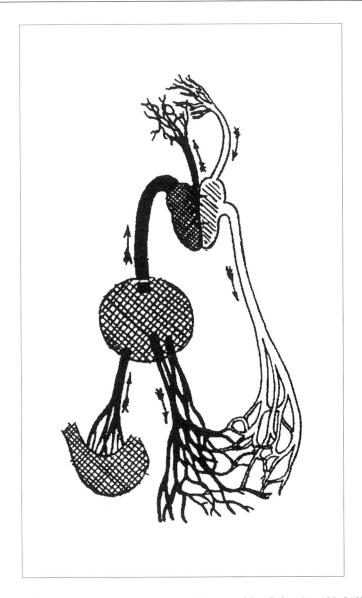

Figure 4 The circulation of the blood as illustrated by Galen (AD 130–210). His concept assumed that there were communications via invisible pores between the two ventricles. The notion was current even after the monumental studies of Vesalius (1514–1564). This view was only finally dispelled with the work of William Harvey (1578–1657) on the circulation of the blood. (Reproduced with permission from Laurence Pollinger (author's agent))

irritating substances leading to fits. This notion was extended to what might now be regarded as 'Jacksonian epilepsy' when the pathological humour was formed in an extremity and travelled to the head. Galen supported this by noting the effect of a tourniquet on the offending part. Toxins were then stopped from reaching the brain, alleviating the condition. A more dramatic method of therapy is also reported – amputation! This prevented viper's toxin from reaching the cerebrum, also being curative.

These views on causation foster a link to the warning signs of attacks, further elucidated by Galen and later Aretaeus[9]. The word 'aura' was taken from the Greek word 'breeze', and in some of the earlier literature is confused with the prodrome, a much longer lasting state. Galen in fact divided the premonitory symptoms into various groups depending on whether they were predominantly sensory, like noises in the head, or psychic, for example slowness of speech. Aretaeus recognized that the aura could commence in parts remote from the brain, including contraction and trembling of the toes and hands, which represented the true aura rather than the more prolonged sensations characteristic of the prodrome. However, apart from more detailed description of the different forms of attacks and the nature of causation, not much was to change for hundreds of years.

EPILEPSY FROM THE BIRTH OF CHRIST TO THE MODERN ERA

After the significant contributions from Greece and the Middle East in the years before Christ, not much new has been added to the under-standing of epilepsy for nearly 2000 years[10]. Medical writers were still active, ringing the changes, annotating, interpreting and occasionally making original observations. The views of the earlier writers were always clearly to the fore. Treatment was rational, if the erroneous views of causation were taken as correct, often concerned with phlegms and humours. Supernatural forces, benign or malevolent were always considered seriously; later, particularly in mediaeval times, astronomical phenomena received attention. The notion of being moon-struck, lunatic and epileptic became interwoven, indeed the popular views that madness and epilepsy were closely linked, still linger to the present time.

Mediaeval times

There were three views about causation of epilepsy; it was due to supernatural forces, humours or irritating and toxic substances.

The idea that supernatural forces caused epilepsy led to entreaties like 'depart demons and go forth ...'. Such statements are recorded quite often in the literature and even today exorcism is practised with hope, and indeed on the part of some, a belief, that it will be successful.

Then there is the question of humours. They were believed to be four in number, blood which was hot and moist, phlegm which was cold and moist, red bile which was hot and dry and finally black bile which was cold and dry. The presence of an imbalance, or the excess of any one humour, could cause seizures. Such notions were totally fanciful but, surprisingly, we still use terms such as 'phlegmatic temperament' which can be seen as calmness verging on the sluggish. In present day parlance perhaps 'laid back' might be an equivalent view. Clearly the concepts of humour have no place in modern physiology though they led to the view that the brain might be starved of air, and anoxic convulsions could result.

Toxins and various irritants were a constant feature of historical texts with the possibility also that infection was important in the causation of attacks. Indeed, according to Lennox[10], Martin Luther, the fervent Protestant reformer, called down all manner of evils on the Catholic Church and these included as well as epilepsy, the plague, syphilis, scurvy, leprosy and carbuncles.

Given this catalogue of causes, rational treatment was clearly impossible. It is, therefore, not surprising that the pharmacopoeia, before the introduction of bromides (see Chapter 3), included such weird potions as powdered human skull, the liver of vultures and mistletoe. Herbal remedies were also highly prized.

Even since the introduction of effective antiepileptic drugs, there remains considerable controversy as to how these now despised treatments from an earlier age relate to current practice, and to medicine of the so-called primitive tribes of the present day. Indeed in Third World countries where resources for the purchase of phar-maceuticals and the training of medical, nursing and paramedical personnel is very limited, traditional healers continue to thrive with their potions, largely made from local, naturally available materials.

There has even been a recent surge of interest in the work of traditional practitioners, from physicians and pharmacologists of developed countries, who have begun to perceive that the drugs used, have, in numerical terms at least, significant importance for many parts of the world. It is possible in addition that some of these folk remedies, if sufficiently researched, might prove to be of value world-wide. There is, unexpectedly, considerable pharmacological study of these compounds in the countries where they are used. Could they come to be incorporated into standard medical practice?

A RECENT SYMPOSIUM

To explore this, a recent symposium was held[11]. It reports surveys carried out in many countries, China, India and African states as well as areas of South America, in relation to traditional practice and medicines used. This revealed perhaps surprisingly little attention to epilepsy, although the condition has no geographical limits. Further, though many of the compounds employed by traditional practitioners have effects on the central nervous system, few have anticonvulsant action. They can be effective as sedatives or hypnotics, and some have anxiolytic properties; Bramim used in India is an exception. It has these actions as well as apparently being an antiepileptic.

Also of interest are some of the concepts applied, for example, the yin and yang (see above). The yin is the female, interior, cold and hypofunctioning principle, whilst the yang has a masculine exterior, heat and hyperfunction effect. These notions are not far removed from those held in ancient times by physicians in Greece and the Middle East, discussed earlier.

It is also intriguing that in this traditional medical practice many of the agents are given to promote positive health rather than to cure disease. The most well-known of these compounds, now beginning to be used fairly widely in the West, is ginseng. It apparently replenishes and supplements vital energy and 'pacifies the spirit'.

Ganoderma is a compound in the therapeutic armamentarium of the traditional Chinese practitioners. Unexpectedly to Western ears, it has been tested widely on animals and shown to have actions on the cardiovascular and respiratory systems. Another action is to prolong phenobarbitone-induced sleeping time, and in mice it protects from

32

nicotine-induced convulsions and death. It is feasible that some anticonvulsant substances, effective in man, may emerge from these studies to supplement the 'accepted' pharmacopoeia.

It may seem strange that neither within the mainstream of medicine nor in the 'traditional' realm was there an effective compound like potassium bromide, the subject of the next chapter.

REFERENCES

1. Singer, C. and Underwood, G.A. (1962). *A Short History of Medicine*. (Oxford, UK: Clarendon Press)
2. Wilson-Kinnier, J.V. and Reynolds, E.H. (1990). Translation and analysis of a cuneiform text forming part of a Babylonian treatise on epilepsy. *Medical History*, **34**, 185
3. Lloyd, G.E.R. (ed.) (1978). *Hippocratic Writings*. Translated by Chadwick, J. and Mann, D. (Harmondsworth, UK: Penguin Books)
4. Janz, D. (1962). The grand mal epilepsies and the sleeping-waking cycle. *Epilepsia*, **3**, 69
5. Bharucha, E.P. and Bharucha, N.E. (1989). Epilepsy in ancient Indian medicine. In Rose, F.C. (ed.) Neuroscience across the centuries. (London: Smith–Gordon)
6. Lai Chi-Wan, L. and Lai Yen-Huei, C. (1991). History of epilepsy in Chinese traditional medicine. *Epilepsia*, **32**, 299
7. Yang Meng Lan. (1983). *Bgi Bing Zhong Yi Zi Wo Liao Yang Quon Shu: Dian Xian*. Beijing, China: Ren Min Wei Sheng Chu Ban She, 29–30
8. Locock, C. (1857). Discussion of paper by E.H. Sieveking. Analysis of fifty two cases of epilepsy observed by the author. *Lancet*, **1**, 527
9. Temkin, O. (1945). *The Falling Sickness*. (Baltimore: Johns Hopkins Press). (2nd edn. 1971, New York: Dover)
10. Lennox, W.G. (1960). *Epilepsy and Convulsive Disorders*. (Boston: Little Brown)
11. Wagner, H. and Vandsworth, M.R. (1990). *Economic and Medical Plant Research. Plants and Traditional Medicines*. (London: Academic Press)

3

Bromides – the beginning of medical treatment

The introduction of bromides into the treatment of epilepsy had quite a different background to what had appertained in the dark age of therapy that stretched from ancient times almost to the 19th century. The ideas of supernatural causation had been swept aside through dissection and experimentation, so that anatomy and physiology were much better understood. There were many along the way who contributed to this growth in knowledge, Thomas Willis (1621–1673), for example, being of great importance. It was he who coined the term 'neurologie'[1].

By the middle of the 19th century there were many famous figures who advanced the understanding of neurology in general, and especially of all aspects of epilepsy. In France at the Salpêtrière there was the distinguished physician, Charcot (1825–1893), among many others, while in England, notably at the National Hospital for the Paralysed and Epileptic and The London Hospital, was Hughlings Jackson (1835–1911) (see Figures 1 and 2). He wrote on neurological topics, and in his selected works[2] one of the two volumes is devoted to epilepsy. Jackson appreciated that seizures need not necessarily be motor, and in fact could be sensory in type. These observations were confirmed by contemporary experimental physiological studies, notably those of Fritsch and Hitzig[3].

Jackson's contributions are most singular in relation to temporal lobe epilepsy. He appreciated and delineated the great variety of clinical manifestations, which did not receive physiological support until after the discovery of electroencephalography some 60 years later. He was also concerned with the total organization of the nervous system into what he termed 'hierarchies'[4]. Lowest level seizures were

35

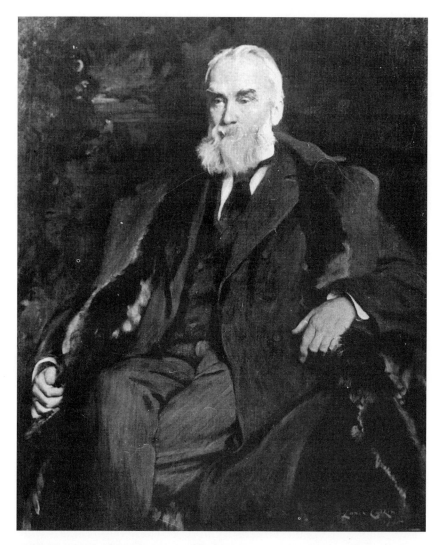

Figure 1 Dr Hughlings Jackson, FRS. Physician to the London Hospital and the National Hospital, Queen's Square. (Reproduced by kind permission of the Archivist of the Royal London Hospital Trust)

described as 'ponto-bulbar'. Middle level fits, associated with the motor cortex and corpus striatum, he described as 'epileptiform'. These unilateral seizures were subsequently known by the term 'focal' or 'partial', while highest level seizures, which Jackson regarded as

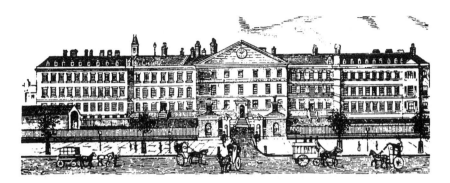

Figure 2   The London Hospital in the 1880s where Hughlings Jackson worked at that time, contemporary with the surgeon Sir Frederick Treves, who was the benefactor of the 'Elephant Man' and introduced an operation for appendicitis. (Reproduced by kind permission of the Archivist of the Royal London Hospital Trust)

'epilepsy proper', would now be called 'generalized'. His most remembered and significant contribution was the neurophysiological definition of epilepsy: 'the name for occasional, sudden, excessive, rapid and local discharges of grey matter'[5]. The growth in knowledge and appreciation of underlying mechanisms paralleled the advances in medical treatment.

THERAPY IN THE MID-NINETEENTH CENTURY

The state of medical treatment of epilepsy in the middle of the nineteenth century is well summarized by the neurologist, Sieveking:

'There is scarcely a substance in the world capable of passing through the gullet of a man that has not at one time or another enjoyed the reputation of being anti-epileptic.'

Nevertheless, there had been attempts to make systematic studies of various therapeutic techniques. Esquirol (1772–1840) at the Salpêtrière[7], submitted 30 patients to a series of treatments in order to study their effectiveness. These included blood lettings, cathartics, baths, cauterization and a variety of medicaments. The patients were carefully prepared for these studies, apparently being promised that cure was certain. There was no difference between the various remedies, but each led to the control of the attacks for a few weeks to a few months. Clearly this is the phenomenon frequently observed to the present day in almost all fields of medicine – the 'placebo' effect. However this term usually shrouds ignorance rather than clarifies the issue.

Other studies were less detailed than Esquirol's, and used the whole gamut of natural remedies. Mistletoe was favoured by some, and there was in the first half of the nineteenth century an interest in the use of simple inorganic compounds such as silver nitrate and zinc oxide, both of which had little effect. Yet it was the simple substance, potassium bromide, which was to prove successful.

When the effects of bromide were first presented by Locock[8] in 1857, the importance of sexual matters was a point for discussion. It had been and continued to be, a matter of concern for the rest of the century, in particular the significance of masturbation.

ONANISM

Onanism, masturbation or self-abuse are different words for the same thing and were regarded as an important cause, not just of epilepsy but of mental illness in general. The history of these ideas was thoroughly discussed by Hare[9] under the heading 'Masturbatory Insanity'. The notion persisted after the introduction of bromides. Indeed Gowers considered this matter at some length in his book on epilepsy and convulsive disorders, published in 1881[10].

> 'Many circumstances render it very difficult to determine the influence of masturbation as a cause of epilepsy. The habit is common in epileptic boys, as in others, but we cannot infer that, in all such cases, it is the cause of the disease. The etiological relation can only be regarded as established when the arrest of the habit, as by circumcision, arrests the disease. But the converse is not true; the continuance of the disease after the arrest of the practice does not disprove the relationship, because, when the 'convulsive habit' is established, it frequently persists after its cause has ceased to be effective. Moreover, in private, it is often difficult to ascertain the existence of the practice, for it is remarkable how long it may elude the observation of friends. It is usually denied by the patient, and the very enquiry renders its

discovery more difficult by suggesting the necessity for concealment. I am inclined to think that it is much less frequently a cause of true epilepsy than of untypical attacks, sometimes hysteroid, sometimes of characters intermediate between hysteroid and epileptoid form. I have so frequently in boys met with this form of attack in association with the practice, that I can scarcely doubt their etiological connection.'

The wide variety of disorders caused by self-abuse can be seen in the following quotation cited by Hare[9]. It is from 'Medical Inquiries Upon Diseases of the Mind' by Benjamin Rush, Professor of Medicine at Philadelphia. Published in 1812, it is the first textbook of psychiatry by an American. Rush mentions onanism as one of the causes of madness.

'Four cases of madness occurred, in my practice, from this cause between the years 1804 and 1807. It is induced more frequently by this cause in young men than is commonly supposed by parents and physicians. Four cases in as many years does not sound too serious, but the morbid effects of intemperance in sexual intercourse with women are feeble and of a transient nature compared with the train of physical and moral evils which this solitary vice fixed upon the body and mind and onanism (excessive or not) produces seminal weakness, impotence, dysury, tabes, dorsalis, pulmonary consumption, dyspepsia, dimness of sight, vertigo, epilepsy, hypochondriasis, loss of memory, manalgia, fatuity and death.'

A great variety of authors at this time, both from this country and on the Continent of Europe, regarded masturbation as a vice which was a frequent cause of insanity. The theoretical basis was that blood was drained from the brain to the body, leading to insanity. Others, however, believed that the reverse occurred, namely that the brain was congested as a result of the act. The various disorders listed as caused by the practice were numerous, but hysterical attacks, epilepsy and convulsions figure prominently.

During the latter part of the 19th century there was a decline in the view that masturbation was an important cause of insanity and epilepsy, but it is interesting that this background of concern about sexual activity was to be of supreme importance in the introduction of bromides.

As Hare[9] points out, psychiatrists and physicians in general were misguided in their views on causation but this did not stop them applying what they saw as appropriate therapeutic measures. These, though encompassing medical means, also included the surgical procedure of castration. Reports of improvement following this operation were used to bolster the incorrect assumptions concerning etiology. The question remains of course, are we nowadays immune to such misguided notions which lead to the application of inappropriate therapy?

SIR CHARLES LOCOCK AND BROMIDES

The year was 1857 and the occasion a presentation by Edward Sieveking (1816–1904) of a paper entitled 'Analysis of 52 cases of epilepsy observed by the author'[11]. It was a discussion after this presentation (Figure 3) that was to prove of greatest importance. Sieveking's paper analyzed the effect of 15 remedies that he had tried, including medications such as antimony, digitalis and silver nitrate. In discussion Sir Charles Locock (1799–1875) made three points[8]. The first concerned crowded teeth. He believed that this was not important in all cases of epilepsy, but in some removal of teeth could effect a cure. Secondly he noted that the practice of onanism was a frequent cause of epilepsy. He felt that this was on the increase and had been overlooked in many instances. The third, the crucial observation, concerned hysterical epilepsy in relation to the menstrual period. Locock had reported that treatment with potassium bromide had been successful in 14 out of 15 cases. It should be emphasized at this point that Sir Charles Locock (see Figure 4) was an obstetrician and was responsible for delivering Queen Victoria's offspring. In spite of these onerous duties and a successful practice in general, he made various observations on convulsions, and quite why he employed potassium bromide for the treatment of his hysterical cases is not fully known. It is our present concern. As Joynt[12] puts it:

'Like many advances in science a chance association was noted by a perceptive individual. Also, as in many discoveries, the reason was wrong but the results were rewarding.'

Joynt summarizes the matter as follows:

Medical Societies.

ROYAL MEDICAL & CHIRURGICAL SOCIETY.

TUESDAY, MAY 11TH, 1857.

SIR C. LOCOCK, PRESIDENT, IN THE CHAIR.

ANALYSIS OF FIFTY-TWO CASES OF EPILEPSY OBSERVED BY THE
AUTHOR.

BY EDWARD H. SIEVEKING, M.D., F.R.C.P.,

PHYSICIAN TO THE LATE DUKE OF CAMBRIDGE, LECTURER ON MATERIA MEDICA
AT, AND ASSISTANT-PHYSICIAN TO, ST. MARY'S HOSPITAL.

Figure 3 Report of the meeting, published in the Lancet, at which, in the discussion following Edward Sieveking's paper, Sir Charles Locock introduced the use of potassium bromide in the treatment of epilepsy

'There was a form also of hysterical epilepsy connected with the menstrual period, and as periodic as that function. This form of the disease was very difficult to treat. The attacks only occurred during the catamenial period, except under otherwise strong exciting causes. He had been baffled in every way in the treatment of this affliction. Some years since, however, he had read in the 'British and Foreign Review' an account of some experiments performed by a German on himself with bromide of potassium. The experimenter had found that when he took ten grains of the preparation, three times a day for fourteen days, it produced temporary impotency, the virile powers returning after leaving off the medicine. He (Dr Locock) determined to try this remedy in cases of hysteria in young women, unaccompanied by epilepsy. He had found it, in doses from five to ten grains, three times a day, of the greatest service. In a case of hysterical epilepsy which had occurred every month for nine years, and had resisted every kind of treatment, he had administered the bromide of potassium. He commenced this

41

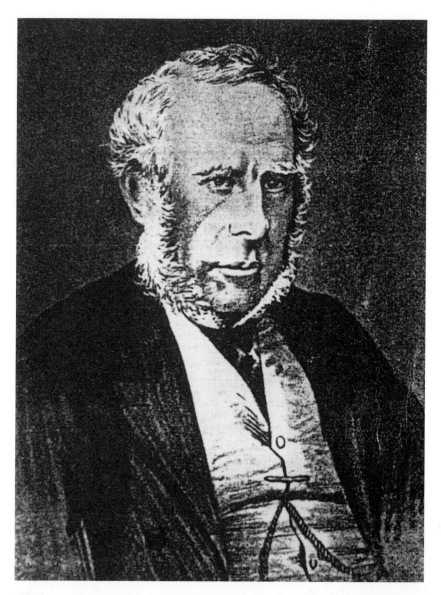

Figure 4 Photograph of Sir Charles Locock (original source unknown). (Reprinted with permission from the *New England Journal of Medicine*, 1957, **256**, p.887)

treatment about fourteen months since. For three months he gave ten grains of the potassium three times a day. He then gave the same dose three times a day for fourteen days before the menstrual period, and latterly had only ordered it in the same dose, three times a day, for a week before the expected catamenia. This patient had had no epilepsy.'

Joynt goes on to say that it was equally effective in 14 out of 15 other cases.

There is some doubt as to where Charles Locock had read the original account of self-induced impotence by bromide, but Joynt found an article by Huette in The Medical Gazette of Paris, 1850[13], which he quotes in translation as follows:

'"the bromide possessed also remarkable power in inducing torpidity of the genital (sic) organs. A patient tormented by a vivid imagination, and subject to frequent consequent pollutions, found himself quite freed from his infirmity after having taken 16 gains per diem for three days; while some patients to whom the drug was administered reproached the author with this effect, which however passes off in a few days after discontinuance of the medicine. The medicine thus seems indicated in chordee, in relieving which camphor and opium so often fail, as also in certain forms of spermatorrhea."

The original article appeared in the Gazette Médicale in which Huette discusses several other uses for potassium bromide. No other reference to this property of bromides was found in the British and Foreign (Medicochirurgical) Review[14], dating from 1857 back to its inception as the British and Foreign Medical Review in 1836.'

Perhaps sadly Locock did not make further advances in the treatment of epilepsy, which had so far been almost entirely by chance. He nevertheless was a man of extremely wide interests, having written his doctoral thesis in 1821 on the use of the stethoscope[15]. Subsequently, his interest in seizures was underlined by the fact that he wrote chapters on infantile convulsions and puerperal convulsions in the 'Cyclopedia of Practical Medicine'[16] which was published in 1833.

However, Lennox, writing in 1957 on 'The Centenary of Bromides'[17] observes that the remarks of Locock 'caused no stampede of science reporters to the telephone'. Perhaps it was because for 2000 years or more doctors had been reporting cures for epilepsy. Yet the same issue of *The Lancet* carried an account of the success of Dr William O'Connor, who had found that the iodide of potassium had relieved both the amenorrhoea and the convulsions of female epileptic patients. Could the readers of this issue of *The Lancet* have concluded that potassium rather than bromide accounted for Locock's success?

SUBSEQUENT INTEREST IN BROMIDES

Dr Edward Sieveking the neurologist, whose presentation sparked the comments by Locock, published two editions of his book '*On Epilepsy and Epileptiform Seizures: Their Causes, Pathology and Treatment*' in 1858 and 1861[6]. In the second and enlarged edition he still wrote about the therapeutic effects of mistletoe but adds:

'however it may be suited to provide good feeling and jocularity at our Christmas games, it has not, in my hands, proved to exert the slightest influence over the epileptic paroxysm.'

Surprisingly only one of the 66 pages on the treatment of epilepsy was given over to the use of bromides. However, notably, he does observe as follows:

'though I have not enjoyed the same amount of success I have found it decidedly beneficial. In one case where the irritation of sexual apparatus was very marked a permanent cure seemed to be attributable to it.'

Locock did not follow his remarks by any publications on bromides, but Radcliffe in his book on convulsions, published in 1861, observed 'I can testify after repeated trials that bromide is often a very valuable remedy in cases where there is not the slightest sign of erotic disposition...'[18]. Radcliffe also observes that 'the name of Sir Charles Locock ought to be remembered with gratitude by every epileptic'.

There is no doubt that his contemporaries appreciated his powers of observation and his voracious appetite for knowledge. Sir James Paget in his obituary on Locock made the following observation as cited by Joynt[12].

'Fortunately Locock made an observation that depended on an acquisitive mind. He gathered knowledge from all quarters, from the honest and the dishonest, from high and low, if only he thought that it was knowledge that he could do good with, he cared little from whence it came.'

FURTHER REPORTS ON POTASSIUM BROMIDE

In 1861 Wilks (1824–1911), a contemporary of Jackson, published his findings on a group of patients treated with bromide[19]. This was apparently the first report of a series of patients. He later, with a certain lack of modesty, stated the belief that this account of his cases treated by potassium bromide was largely responsible for the drug's being so widely employed subsequently. He also remarked that the results were much more effective than he had anticipated. The dose generally used appears to have been 5–10 grains, three times a day, but there still seems to have been doubt in the minds of the physicians of the time, even Locock himself, as to whether it was the potassium rather than the bromide that was the effective element, in spite of the fact that potassium iodide had been used for other conditions but was found to be inactive for epilepsy.

At The National Hospital for the Paralysed and Epileptic, later to become The Hospital for Nervous Diseases, Drs Ramskill in 1863[20] and Radcliffe in 1861[18] both employed bromides, as did Hughlings Jackson. Interestingly he combined digitalis with bromide in the treatment of many patients. Digitalis was a therapy for epilepsy that had been introduced much earlier by the physician Parkinson (1755–1824), and its use lingered into the bromide era, according to Gowers[10], although Hughlings Jackson reported that in certain cases, such as those of brain tumour, digitalis did not seem to be a useful addition to the bromide therapy.

Belgrave showed in 1865 that bromides were effective in the treatment of insanity, including epilepsy[21], and in the same year Crighton-Browne, practising in Scotland, also indicated that it was efficacious. Not everyone, however, found it valuable and the matter was complicated by the fact that when it was withdrawn seizures became even more severe. Indeed, Hughlings Jackson by 1870 had already warned that when it was decided to abandon treatment, gradual reduction of the dosage was essential[22].

BROMIDES AFTER LOCOCK

In his book on epilepsy, published in 1881, Gowers[10] devotes 19 pages to the use of bromides for epilepsy (Figures 5 and 6). It is of interest, however, that he deals with other forms of treatment which we now know are of negligible value. He mentions that zinc possibly deserves some of the repute as a remedy for epilepsy that it had enjoyed for more than 100 years. He cites one particular patient's history, commenting that zinc is capable of producing just the same effects as bromide. In this 20-year-old woman no fits occurred for a 9-month period. He also adds that the addition of arsenic to bromide did not produce any marked benefit in his experience.

Regarding the use of iron Gowers observes that: 'certain distinguished authorities as Brown-Séquard and Hughlings Jackson, have discounted the administration of iron to epileptics, asserting that while it improves the health of epileptics, it increases the frequency and severity of fits'.

He comments that chloral hydrate, either alone or in combination with bromide or other remedies, has had little benefit, although in the past it has enjoyed 'a high repute'. Gowers states 'I have seen, in a few cases in which I have tried them, no resulting benefit'.

Trephining (see Chapter 5) is also given attention by Gowers. He comments:

'A very old remedy for epilepsy, has lately been again brought into prominence in consequence of the more exact localization of diseases of the brain which furnish the surgeon with a more accurate locality for operation.'

Before Gowers deals with the first aid treatment of seizures, there is a brief paragraph on castration. We have already discussed the question of sexual activity, and it is of course curious that the first real breakthrough came when, quite wrongly, the association was made between sex and epilepsy. In relation to castration Gowers observes:

'it has been proposed as a remedial measure, and has been performed without effect. It has been lately revived by Bacon[23] as a means of arresting epilepsy due to masturbation in adult insane patients.'

EPILEPSY

AND OTHER

CHRONIC CONVULSIVE DISEASES:

THEIR CAUSES, SYMPTOMS, & TREATMENT

BY

W. R. GOWERS, M.D., F.R.C.P.

ASSISTANT PROFESSOR OF CLINICAL MEDICINE IN UNIVERSITY COLLEGE ;
SENIOR ASSISTANT PHYSICIAN TO UNIVERSITY COLLEGE HOSPITAL ;
PHYSICIAN TO THE NATIONAL HOSPITAL FOR THE PARALYSED AND EPILEPTIC.

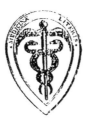

LONDON :

J. & A. CHURCHILL, NEW BURLINGTON STREET.

1881.

Figure 5 Title page of book on epilepsy by William Gowers (1845–1915), which contains a short section on bromides, as well as many other remedies that had been tried, but not yet discarded, by practising physicians [10]

BY THE SAME AUTHOR.

A MANUAL AND ATLAS OF MEDICAL
OPHTHALMOSCOPY. With Sixteen Coloured,
Autotype, and Lithographic Plates. 8vo. price 18s.

PSEUDO-HYPERTROPHIC MUSCULAR
PARALYSIS; a Clinical Lecture. With Illustrations. 8vo. price 3s. 6d.

THE DIAGNOSIS OF DISEASES OF
THE SPINAL CORD. Second Edition. 8vo.
With Illustrations. Price 4s. 6d.

Preparing for publication.

A MANUAL OF DISEASES OF THE
NERVOUS SYSTEM. For Students and Practitioners.

Figure 6 Gowers' wide range of neurological interests is indicated by this note of his other publications, taken from his book on epilepsy

He mentions a less drastic measure in boys – circumcision – which he regards as usually successful, at least in the cases where there was reason to associate epilepsy with masturbation.

EARLY STATISTICAL APPROACHES

Gowers begins his chapter on treatment with general observations on the evaluation of treatment and some of these remain helpful today. He notes that a large number of cases are under observation for too short a time to enable the effect of the remedies to be fully estimated, and of the cases in which benefit is derived, there is no means of assessing how many relapse when treatment is discontinued. His figures on 562 patients are of interest, because he reports that of these, 241 were fit-free under the period of observation, and some apparently had discontinued treatment but remained seizure-free. In 266 cases improvement occurred, the frequency of attacks being reduced in many to one-thirtieth, one-fiftieth and even one-hundredth of their former frequency. There was a residuum of about ten percent in whom no improvement occurred by any method of treatment. This is of considerable importance because it is generally still accepted, even with modern treatment, that about this proportion of patients fail to gain any benefit. Gowers warns us that:

'indications for special treatment in epilepsy is a subject of greatest importance. There is no point in therapeutics however more open to fallacy, or on which more generalizations have been published, which subsequent observation has proved inaccurate.'

He begins his section on bromides by indicating that this compound has 'almost' superseded other drugs in the treatment of the disease. He states:

'the single benefit which, in the majority of cases attends its use, has rendered the administration of bromides in the treatment of epilepsy almost equivalent expressions.'

The question of cure versus relapse of the symptoms next occupies his thoughts. He observes that the cessation of treatment and the relapse that occurs indicates that cure has not been effected. Gowers emphasizes that a search for remedies with a more permanent effect must obviously be continued, but clearly feels that this is not an overall objection to the treatment with bromides.

All the problems that still beset those who treat patients with epilepsy receive Gowers' attention. His observations cover both the question of compliance and titrating of the individual patient's dosage so it remains below a toxic level. He also notes that if non-compliance occurs and relapse results, reinstating the treatment is usually effective. He also warns that bromides 'should never be suddenly left off'.

The case histories cited testify to the value of treatment. The methods of administration and the dosage are considered in detail.

He recommends 5 or 10 grains per day. Gowers warns that continued administration of 60–120 grains invariably leads to bromism which he defines as physical feebleness and mental dullness. Sometimes this can amount to a semi-imbecile condition with drooling speech and a dribbling mouth. He also observes on the positive side that for some patients, when treatment with bromide is given and cessation of fits occurs, there is an improvement in their mental power.

The side-effect that he mentions particularly is acne. There is, in his experience, a matter of individual idiosyncrasy as some patients take large doses daily for years without any sign of dermatological problems, while others develop them quite speedily. The acne could be extremely severe with large painful pustules resulting in considerable permanent disfigurement with pitting, reddening and thickening of the skin.

OTHER TREATMENTS

Of considerable interest is Gowers' comment on the use of digitalis. It was a very old remedy for epilepsy recommended as long ago as 1640 by Parkinson and particularly popular in the West of England. Digitalis could lead to decrease in frequency of attacks and sometimes arrest for short periods in some patients. Todd[24] thought that nocturnal epilepsy was especially associated with cardiac disease, while Gowers observed that patients with heart disease may only have attacks by day.

Perhaps the most surprising observation is the use of cannabis. Gowers observes: 'it is of small value as an adjunct to bromide, but is sometimes of considerable service given separately'.

RECENT USE OF BROMIDES

'The use of bromides for the treatment of epilepsy is over 100 years old. It is unusual that a drug with any specificity was extant at that time, with the notable exceptions of digitalis, quinine, and a few others. It is also unusual that a drug with this lifespan is still used; not having been supplanted by treatments devised with modern methods of drug manufacture'[12].

Joynt further observes that: 'I suspect that there are very few working in the field of epilepsy that have much direct experience of bromides.' I can concur with this statement, having only seen one case at the beginning of my interest in the subject some 25 years ago, and have never prescribed it personally. Nevertheless as late as 1963 Haddow Keith [25] in his textbook *'Convulsive Disorders in Children'* (a book notable for a long section on the ketogenic diet, see Chapter 5, whose use is also virtually extinct) has, in the chapter on antiepileptic medication, a section devoted to the use of bromides which is almost as long as that for barbiturates. He comments 'although other drugs have been developed, bromides remain among the most effective anticonvulsant medications'.

However it is the much earlier work of Aldren Turner [26], published in 1907 in a book entitled *'Epilepsy – a Study of the Idiopathic Disease'*, which gives the most detailed and comprehensive view of the outcome of treatment with bromides. The findings, which compare with those of other contemporary physicians, act as basic information about the type of treatment outcome that can be expected (Figure 7), with about a quarter of cases 'arrested' and a further, slightly larger, number who show improvement.

OTHER ASPECTS OF EPILEPSY

While Gowers and his neurological colleagues such as Aldren Turner were continuing to make progress in the treatment of epilepsy, there were physicians pushing forward the frontiers of other aspects of neurology and considering attack disorders in a wider context. Gowers himself had been interested in what he called 'The Border-lands of Epilepsy'. The book with this title was finally published in 1907 towards the end of his life [27]. It dealt with faints, vasovagal attacks, vertigo, migraine and sleep disorders. He also added views on their treatment; recommendations involved arsenic, quinine and strychnine, coupled with exercise and open air! Clearly Gowers' forte was in the diagnostic field. He set out lists of differences between hysteria and epilepsy which are still of value now when the distinction has to be made between genuine and pseudo-seizures [28].

At the same time in Paris, at the Salpêtrière, Charcot was working on this theme, as was at that time a notable neurologist, none other *showing the general results of prolonged bromide medication in 366 cases treated at the Queen Square Hospital.*

Cases of arrest - - - -	86 or 23·5	per cent.
Cases showing improvement -	105 or 28·7	„
Confirmed cases - - -	175 or 47·8	„
TOTALS - -	366 100	„

These figures are in general harmony with the observations of some other writers on the subject, notably Binswanger,[1] who refers to the result of bromide treatment in the Stephansfeld Institute for Epileptics in the following table, although the total number of cases on which the observations were made is not stated :

Arrest of seizures during treatment -	23·3 per cent.
Diminution in frequency to one-half -	40·0 „
No material change - - - -	36·6 „

Figure 7 Page reproduced from W. Aldren Turner's book[25], indicating results of treatment with bromide. It is often cynically stated that there has not been a great overall change in outlook in spite of newer drugs, though certainly side-effects are greatly reduced compared with those produced by prolonged bromide medication

than Freud (1856–1939). Though he was subsequently to be the founder of the school of psychoanalysis, his background in physiology and neurology was thorough. He also commented on how discoveries were made. Freud thought that it was only necessary simply to stare all the known facts in the face and continue to do so until they fell into place! He also advocated the therapeutic use of cocaine, a matter which has recently produced some negative comments on his overall contribution to psychiatry. Under Charcot in Paris in the mid 1880s Freud studied hypnosis. He was particularly interested in the phenomenon at that stage as he and his collaborator, Breuer, found that this technique could be used in the treatment of patients with 'painful' memories deeply embedded in the subconscious.

Hypnosis had a long history and still remains controversial. It began in the 18th century with Mesmer (1734–1815) and at that time he gave his name to it (Figures 8 and 9). There have been phases of

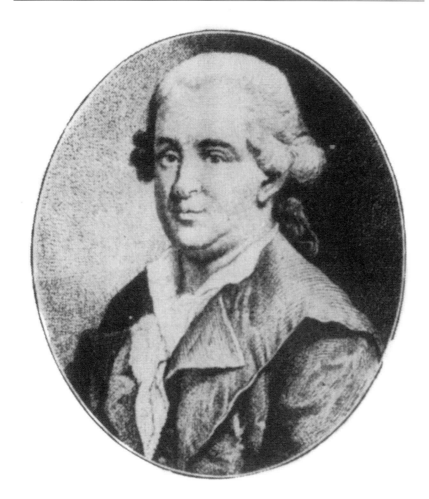

Figure 8 Franz Mesmer, founder of hypnosis in the late eighteenth century. The relationship between hypnosis, hysteria and epilepsy persisted until the end of the 19th century, when the notable neurologist Charcot was involved. (Reproduced with permission from *Hospital Doctor*, 1983. Original source untraced)

interest ever since. In the following century, according to Freud, Charcot first demonstrated that hysterical manifestations whether in the form of epilepsy or, for example, limb paralysis, could be removed or indeed reproduced by hypnosis, thus confirming the psychological origin of such presenting symptoms[29]. Gowers contemporaneously was attempting clearly to separate hysteroid symptoms, hystero-

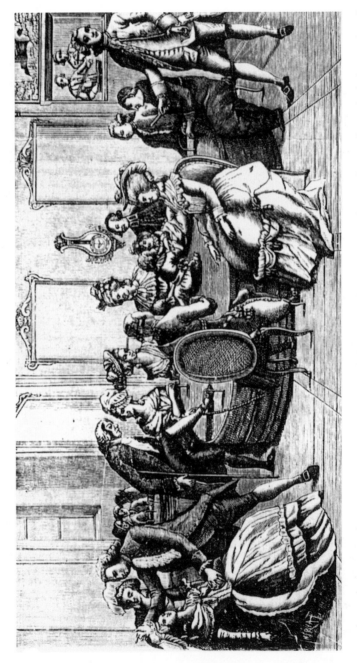

Figure 9 Mesmer used different instruments for inducing trances. This illustration shows a large tub to which the paralysed parts of patients were attached with ropes and hooks, in order to effect treatment. Mesmer made many claims of cure. (Reproduced with permission from *Hospital Doctor*, 1983. Original source untraced)

epilepsy and 'hysteria major', distinguishing these from true epilepsy, whilst Weir Mitchell, the American neurologist, was quite aware of the difficulties of diagnosis[30], as we are still today, in the treatment of disorders which have hysterical concomitants.

CONCLUSION

It is clear that the second half of the nineteenth century was one of great expansion of neurological knowledge in general, and from our point of view, of the medical treatment of epilepsy with bromides. This did, however, introduce us to the condition of status epilepticus as Hunter firmly asserts[31]. That it was a condition to be considered carefully was emphasized by Aldren Turner in 1907 in his book on epilepsy which gives clear evidence on this matter, as well as statistical data on the response to treatment with bromides[26]. His findings are not dissimilar, or so a cynic has suggested, to the use of even the very latest antiepileptic agent in previously drug-resistant patients!

REFERENCES

1. Willis, I. (1685). The London practice of physick. In *The Whole Practical Part of Physick*. (London: George and Crooke)
2. Taylor, J. (1931/32). *Selected Writings of John Hughlings Jackson, Vols 1 and 2*. (London: Hodder and Stoughton). (Reprinted 1958, New York: Basic Books)
3. Fritsch, G. and Hitzig, E. (1870). Uber die elektrische erregbarkeit grosshirns. *Arch. Anat. Physiol. Med.*, **37**, 300
4. Jackson, J.H. (1890). On convulsive seizures. *Br. Med. J.*, **2**, 703, 765, 821
5. Jackson, J.H. (1873). On the anatomical, physiological and pathological investigations of epilepsies. *West Riding Lunatic Asylum Med. Rep.*, **3**, 315
6. Sieveking, E.H. (1858). *On Epilepsy and Epileptiform Seizures: Their Causes, Pathology and Treatment*. 1st edn. (London: Churchill) (2nd edn. 1861)
7. Temkin, O. (1945). *The Falling Sickness*. (Baltimore: Johns Hopkins Press) (2nd edn., 1971, New York: Dover)
8. Locock, C. (1857). Discussion of paper by E.H. Sieveking. Analysis of fifty-two cases of epilepsy observed by the author. *Lancet*, **1**, 527
9. Hare, E.H. (1962).Masturbatory insanity. *J. Ment. Sci.*, **108**, 1
10. Gowers, W.R. (1881). *Epilepsy and other Chronic Convulsive Diseases: Their*

Causes, Symptoms and Treatment. (London: Churchill)

11. Sieveking, E.H. (1857). Analysis of 52 cases of epilepsy observed by the author. *Lancet*, **1**, 527

12. Joynt, R.J. (1974). The use of bromides for epilepsy. *Am. J. Dis. Child.*, **128**, 362

13. Huette, M. (1850). Recherches sur les properties physiologiques et therapeutiques du bromure de potassium. *Med. Gaz. Paris*, **21**, 432. (See reference 14)

14. Huette, M. (1850). Recherches sur les properties physiologiques et therapeutiques du bromure de potassium. *Br. Foreign Med. Chir. Rev.*, **6**, 556. (See reference 13)

15. Locock, C. (1821). *De Cordis Palpitatione.* (Edinburgh: P. Neill)

16. Locock, C. (1833). Infantile convulsions, puerperal convulsions. In Forbes, J., Tweedy, A. and Conolly, J. (eds.) *The Cyclopedia of Medicine.* (London: Sherwood, Gilbert and Piper, Baldwin and Craddock)

17. Lennox, W.G. (1957). The centenary of bromides. *N. Engl. J. Med.*, **256**, 887

18. Radcliffe, C.B. (1861). *Epileptic and Other Convulsive Affections of the Nervous System, Their Pathology and Treatment.* (3rd edn., London: Churchill) (1st edn. 1854)

19. Wilks, Sir Samuel. (1861). Bromide and iodide of potassium in epilepsy. *Med. Times and Gaz. (Lond.)*, **2**, 1861

20. Ramskill, J.S. (1863). Bromides in epilepsy. *Med. Times and Gaz. (Lond.)*, **2**, 221

21. Belgrave, T.B. (1865). The bromides, of potassium, cadmium and ammonia in the treatment of insanity. *J. Ment. Sci.*, **11**, 363

22. Jackson, J.H. (1870). Digitalis with bromide of potassium in epilepsy. *Br. Med. J.*, **1**, 32

23. Bacon, N. (1880). Castration for treatment of epilepsy. *J. Ment. Sci.*, October, 470

24. Todd, R.B. (1854). Clinical lectures on paralysis. In *Diseases of the Brain and Other Affections of the Nervous System.* (London: Churchill)

25. Keith, Haddow, M. (1963). *Convulsive Disorders in Children with Reference to the Treatment with Ketogenic Diet.* (London: Churchill)

26. Turner, W.A. (1907). *Epilepsy – a Study of the Idiopathic Disease.* (New York: Macmillan). (Reprinted 1973, New York: Raven Press)

27. Gowers, W.R. (1907). *The Borderlands of Epilepsy.* (London: Churchill)

28. Scott, D.F. (1982). Recognition of pseudo-seizures. In Riley, T.L. and Roy, A. (eds.) *Pseudoseizures.* (Baltimore: Williams and Wilkins)

29. Massey, W.E. (1982). History of epilepsy and hysteria. In Riley T.L. and Roy, A. (eds.) *Pseudoseizures.* (Baltimore: Williams and Wilkins)

30. Burr, A. (1929). *Weir Mitchell – His Life and Letters.* (New York: Duffield)

31. Hunter, R.A. (1959/60). Status epilepticus, history, incidence and problems. *Epilepsia*, **1**, 162

4

Phenobarbitone – the first fruit of synthetic chemistry

Controversy has perhaps surprisingly occupied a great deal of the history of chemistry. In mediaeval times there were at least two contentious matters, the first was the search for an elixir of life, the second, with which the alchemist also struggled for centuries, was the attempt to produce gold from base metals. These efforts came to nothing but even later, in the eighteenth century, chemistry was not devoid of controversy. Perhaps the most notable was the question of combustion and the existence of 'phlogiston'. It was only when oxygen was discovered that this mysterious substance could be deleted from the language of chemists.

The next matter to cause concern was whether or not it was possible to make naturally occurring substances from 'pure' chemicals. When Wöhler showed by his synthesis of urea that this was possible, he allowed organic chemistry to begin and flourish in the way we know today.

We must not deny, however, that luck, chance and serendipity played a considerable part. It remains uncertain which of these aspects of discovery was involved in formulating the concept of the benzene ring, the essential component of many organic compounds. The honours must go to Kékulé (1829–1896), a notable German organic chemist, who put forward views on the benzene ring structure.

This monumental discovery, according to Mavromatis[1], occurred in hypnagogia, a unique state of consciousness between wakefulness and sleep, where a variety of mental phenomena may occur, both normal and abnormal, including creativity. Kékulé's observations have been called 'the most brilliant piece of prediction to be found in the whole range of organic chemistry'.

It was reported in 1890 to the German Chemical Society. Apparently he, dozing on a bus, saw atoms gambolling before his eyes. On returning home Kékulé spent most of the night sketching the various forms he remembered; he had learnt the trick of using the state of hypnagogia with startling results. Another account is also given[2]:

'I was sitting writing at my textbook; but the work did not progress; my thoughts were elsewhere. I turned my chair to the fire and dozed. Again the atoms were gambolling before my eyes. This time the smaller groups kept modestly in the background. My mental eyes, rendered more acute by repeated visions of the kind, could now distinguish larger structures, of manifold conformation: long rows, sometimes more closely fitted together; all twining and twisting in snakelike motion. But look! What was that? One of the snakes had seized hold of its own tail, and the form whirled mockingly before my eyes. As if by a flash of lightning I awoke; and this time also I spent the rest of the night working out the consequences of the hypothesis.'

THE FIRST BREAKTHROUGH

The benzene ring to which Kékulé applied this image is a stable structure, yet the bonding of the atoms themselves appears to be a dynamic process. With this remarkable new notion, chemistry could again progress, and from the thousands of compounds obtained it was possible to screen those with a therapeutic action. Nearly a century after Wöhler synthesized urea, phenobarbitone became available for the treatment of epilepsy. It was the first example of a synthetic chemical to be used in this way, and the year was 1912.

Obviously from the synthesis of a molecule to the appearance of the compound on the pharmacy shelves, represents not only an enormous financial cost, but also a considerable time lag. For phenobarbitone it was only a few years, but for some compounds a much longer latency occurs (see subsequent chapters).

THE BARBITURATES

The synthesis of barbituric acid, from which the whole line of sedative and hypnotic drugs derived, occurred on Saint Barbara's day in 1864, hence the name. It was nearly 70 years later in 1912 that the clinical use of phenobarbitone was first put forward by Hauptmann. Exactly how he made the discovery of the antiepileptic action is uncertain, but the fact that bromides were sedative was clearly an important factor. Extracts from a translation of his initial article reveal something of how his findings came about.

BARBITURATES AS SEDATIVES

Dr Alfred Hauptmann begins his monumental article (Figure 1) on the 'use of phenobarbitone in the treatment of epilepsy' by dealing with the soporific effects of barbiturates[3]. In particular he says, up to this point our experience adds nothing new to previous knowledge. He writes:

> 'In the course of the last few weeks a great many articles have appeared dealing with the results achieved with the new soporific 'Luminal', (by Farbwerke Fr. Bayer and Co.), detailing its outstanding usefulness as a soporific, a sedative and an hypnotic since, in the form of soluble sodium salt, it can also be used subcutaneously. To report further on what we have already said on this subject would not result in anything contradictory.'

27. August 1912.   MUENCHENER MEDIZINISCHE WOCHENSCHRIFT.   1907

In diese Gruppe möchte ich auch jene Individuen einbeziehen, die teils durch ihren Beruf (Kesselschmiede, Schlosser etc.), teils durch überstandene Noxen (Trauma, Typhus etc.) Veränderungen ihres nervösen Kochlearapparates zeigen.

C. Otosklerose.

Ob die Veränderungen des Gehörorganes, die man als Otosklerose bezeichnet, in das Mittelohr oder in das innere Ohr oder in beide zu lokalisieren sind, ist eine Frage, auf die an dieser Stelle nicht weiter eingegangen werden soll. Es ist aber ausser Zweifel, dass die nervösen Elemente des Ohres in einer Reihe von Fällen sicher in den pathologischen Prozess einbezogen sind.

Ausserdem spricht das familiäre Auftreten und die Heredität dieser Erkrankung dafür, dass es sich bei solchen Individuen um ein a priori nicht normales, und zwar minderwertiges Gehörorgan handelt, das eine geringere Widerstandsfähigkeit besitzt.

Dieses Faktum allein genügt schon, um bei solchen Individuen die Salvarsanbehandlung zu unterlassen. Bei 2 Fällen von Otosklerose, die ich erst nach der Injektion zur Untersuchung zugewiesen bekam, hatte nach Angabe der Patienten die Schwerhörigkeit seit der Salvarsanbehandlung bedeutend und rapid zugenommen. Beide Kranken behaupteten, vorher normal gehört zu haben. In beiden Fällen fand ich bei voll-

beiden Ohren auf, die seither unverändert blieb. Auch L e i d - l e r hat aus der Wiener Poliklinik einen derartigen Patienten demonstriert.

Ob auf Grund der vorliegenden Beobachtungen bei Lues hereditaria Salvarsan injiziert werden soll, muss eine noch offene Frage bleiben. Denn einerseits sind bedeutende Besserungen, andererseits ebenso bedeutende Verschlechterungen in der Funktionstüchtigkeit des Ohres sichergestellt.

Aus der Psychiatrischen und Nervenklinik ! der Universität Freiburg i. B. (Geheimrat H o c h e).

Luminal bei Epilepsie.

Von Dr. A l f r e d H a u p t m a n n, Assistent der Klinik.

Im Laufe der letzten Wochen ist eine grosse Anzahl von Mitteilungen über die Ergebnisse, welche mit einem neuen Schlafmittel „Luminal" (Farbwerke Fr. Bayer & Co.) erzielt worden sind, erschienen, die insgesamt seine hervorragende Brauchbarkeit als Schlafmittel, Sedativum und Hypnotikum hervorheben, zumal es in Form des löslichen Natriumsalzes auch eine subkutane Anwendung gestattet. Eine ausführliche Mitteilung unserer diesbezüglichen Mitteilungen würde nichts wesentlich Abweichendes ergeben.

Auch wir fanden, dass es in Dosen von 0,2 bis 0,3 ...

Figure 1 The first publication in 1912 on the use of 'Luminal in Epilepsy' by Dr Alfred Hauptmann

So, from the start we get the impression of considerable activity and, presumably, discrepancies between different writers on the efficacy of various other barbiturates and their dosage. Hauptmann continues:

'We, too, have found that dosages of 300–400 mg yield quite good results in insomnia of light to medium degree: Luminal proved successful, but in severe cases of insomnia and states of restlessness and excitation the dosage often had to be increased to 500–600 mg: in these states especially the possibility of subcutaneous application became a most agreeable feature. For cases like this scopolamine had been the only drug available, with its effects often exceeding what was desired, even if administered in small doses (quite apart from its disagreeable and dangerous side effects). It is here that Luminal can fill the so far open gap of a fairly mild sedative with subcutaneous application. In cases of severe excitation its application appears contra-indicated, if for no other reason than certainly because the results only begin to show approximately one hour after administration; Luminal will not be able to compete effectively with scopolamine here.'

One is struck by the marked limitations of the drugs available at the time, and is somewhat amazed by the high dosage recommended. However, bringing us immediately to the point of interest, Dr Hauptmann continues:

'Up to this point our experience adds nothing to previous knowledge. However, I should draw attention to the susceptibility of epilepsy or rather of epileptic attacks through Luminal. This became apparent when using the new medication as a tranquilliser, also with epileptic patients, whereupon I proceeded systematically to use Luminal in severe cases of epilepsy over long periods. To date there has been no mention in the published articles about Luminal of its application in the treatment of epilepsy; at most it had been administered as a sedative for states of epileptic agitation.'

It seems that definite tranquillization was obtained in patients with epilepsy, and he observed for the *first* time that seizures were controlled. This appears to be an example of serendipitous discovery, the importance being that the significance of the observation was recognized, and Dr Hauptmann as we shall see, went on to treat patients with epilepsy, specifically with a view to controlling their seizures. This is certainly an example of chance favouring the prepared mind.

Selection of patients

Dr Hauptmann's comments in the following paragraph are of considerable interest, not least in their sophistication. Many of his observations are still apposite today, particularly as initial reports on response to drugs are hastily presented without adequate attention to background or detail.

'In order not to be misled by variations in the frequency of attacks I limited my observations to cases which had been in our own hospital for several years and thus had the frequency of their attacks recorded meticulously, or patients where exact records made precise comparisons possible. I furthermore believed that my conclusions should be based on research lasting several months, again in order to eliminate errors of random changes in state. We treated almost without exception, very severe cases who had been administered high doses of bromide over long periods of time, even years. It is precisely vis-à-vis these cases who are a constant danger to themselves and to other patients because of repeated attacks several times a day and above all because of their pronounced state of semi-consciousness and excitability, whose state of nutrition and strength deteriorates progressively, whose acne pustules require steadily more frequent surgical intervention, that the search for a different, more powerful and less damaging remedy is justified.'

It is of interest to note how troublesome the skin eruptions related to bromide were. Hauptmann says that some of the newer bromide preparations, though not showing these side-effects to such an extent, are less efficacious in the treatment of the condition.

Clinical observations

Hauptmann's report continues:

'My observations started in mid-February of this year (i.e. 1912).

Naturally, it must be our aim to attain optimum results with the smallest possible dosages of the medicine. Even in the most severe cases I have never had to use more than 300 mg (administered internally in tablet form). Since such a dose naturally already had a sleep-inducing effect it proved expedient to administer it in the evening before bedtime, or split it into part-doses, such as 100 mg in the morning and 200 mg at night. The morning dose of 100 mg did not evoke any sleepiness worth mentioning in any of the patients. I should also emphasize at once that there have never been any complaints about repugnant taste, there has been no incidence of indigestion, no rashes were observed (as mentioned occasionally in medical literature), nor any disorder of pupils, reflexes, hearts, etc.; urine was always free of pathological components. These findings are of prime importance mainly because up until now the remedy has never yet been administered over so prolonged a period of time and because on the part of the manufacturers a cumulative effect had been observed in animals. Despite this continuous dispensing, no harmful side-effects became apparent, cumulation did not occur either, much rather, possibly a certain habituation.'

Hauptmann noted as we do today with many effective medications, that not only the frequency but the nature of the attacks changed.

'The action upon the attacks was twofold: the frequency of the attacks abated appreciably, or attacks stopped altogether in the less severe cases, and the nature of the attacks changed: severe attacks with tonic-clonic spasms, tongue-biting, etc. were replaced by attacks of shorter duration or brief faints: the latter were not long and followed by semi-consciousness, but even after brief impairments of consciousness patients would awake lucidly.'

Illustrative case

Although Hauptmann demurs from presenting many case histories, he does include in his paper one brief history, with an excellent chart of a single patient with especially severe epilepsy, on high doses of bromides for many years, without success (Figure 2).

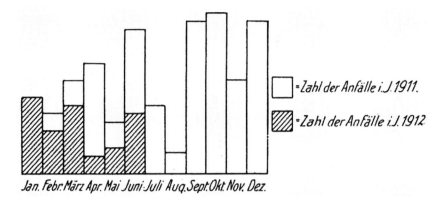

Figure 2   Histogram from the paper of Dr Alfred Hauptmann[3], showing the decrease in fit frequency in one patient when Luminal was substituted for bromide. The open columns show the number of seizures (Anfälle) in 1911, and the hatched columns those in 1912. Observations finished in June of that year. There is a slight increase in that month, probably indicating, as Hauptmann suggests, drug tolerance

'I have chosen this particular case because the data available allow a precise comparison of the number of attacks over the full year. The reduction in the number of attacks from February 1912 shows up clearly, not only in comparison with the latter months of 1911, but also compared with the corresponding months of February to June 1911. But it was not just the number of attacks which subsided (a dosage exceeding 300 mg might even have reduced the number still further), the attacks themselves became much "lighter", states of semi-consciousness, during which the patient had very often inflicted severe injuries upon himself, disappeared almost completely. As a result the psychological state also remained static; although the constant relapses caused by the epileptic process of the brain naturally remained unchanged, the mental agility was nevertheless enhanced. The state of nutrition and strength which had suffered greatly as a result of the administration of bromide over many years improved to a quite extraordinary degree.'

Proof of efficacy

Although the report of Hauptmann does not include the type of sophisticated trial design that we would now expect, it shows quite clearly that Luminal was effective in that chronically institutionalized patients were able to leave and resume their occupations. Compliance with medication was also emphasized.

'When I spoke about less severe cases, where the attacks stopped altogether, this only included the mildest among the more serious cases, i.e. still within the category where bromide would hardly have any effect; all were patients who, because of the number and severity of their attacks, had to be detained in a secure institution. These cases could – through administration of Luminal – be brought to the point where they could be discharged, and in some instances could be allowed to resume their occupations, albeit with strict instructions to continue their treatment as prescribed.'

Hauptmann next discusses the question as to whether or not it is better to allow patients to have seizures, because if they do not irritability could occur. His observations correspond to our current experience with the majority of epileptic patients.

'Because, naturally, Luminal is not a cure for epilepsy, it does not specifically influence the epileptic brain process; it is merely capable of reducing the sensitivity of the cerebral cortex and by so doing to stall the attacks. Many authors consider this course as contra-indicated; they feel that the attacks should bring about a "discharge" as it were; the lack of discharge leading to increased irritability. In the patients I have observed so far I never noticed any negative results which could have been a consequence of the missing discharge, in any case the state of agitation did not occur more frequently or more violently than before.'

It was quite clear that the effect of Luminal was not curative, and to check the possibility of long-term effects, what happened when the drug was stopped was also investigated.

'Because prescribing continuously will probably be necessary; deliberate interruption of supplies for several days resulted in immediate increase in frequency of attacks. The same effect is after all common with sudden deprivation of bromide, and it remains to be observed whether Luminal might have a beneficial after-effect, which seems improbable in theory, however.'

Hauptmann's conclusions

'Summarizing my observations, Luminal seems capable of exerting a favourable influence upon epilepsy by reducing the number and severity of attacks. Its range of applications will mainly be with those severest cases of epilepsy which are beyond the power of influence of even the heaviest of bromide dosages. Cases of medium severity can be rendered free of attacks with dosages of 150–200 mg per day; the more severe ones are unlikely to require more than 300 mg. Harmful side-effects have never been observed, not even in continuous daily use over several months; and in particular there was no cumulative effect. Luminal can, therefore, also usefully replace bromide in less severe cases, where the latter's use seems contra-indicated because of its side-effects.'

The article finishes with an indication that Hauptmann regarded his findings as preliminary.

'These conclusions must only be regarded as the preliminary findings of the trial so far, which still have to be extended in respect of both time and number of cases studied.'

HAUPTMANN'S DISCOVERY

Nowadays a report like that of Hauptmann, revealing such an effective treatment in a chronic disorder, would be greeted with ballyhoo. Words such as 'breakthrough' and 'miracle drug' would appear in newspaper headlines, and command considerable attention in other media, perhaps even before the paper was published in a medical journal! This did not happen of course following Hauptmann's 1912 article on the use of Luminal. Yet in spite of the fact that it was published in a German journal, it came to be used widely quite quickly. There was some delay in prescription in the US, but following the end of the First World War in 1918, it quickly became the treatment of choice, with the publication of articles containing significant series of patients showing beneficial results. There was, not unexpectedly, a lingering use of bromides for a considerable time, indeed even after the introduction of phenytoin in 1937.

In the 1970s Coatsworth carried out, for the US National Institutes of Health, an authoritative review of the clinical efficacy of marketed antiepileptic drugs[4]. Phenobarbitone was cited in about 40 papers, only a few less than phenytoin, even though many other compounds had been introduced, including ethotoin, phenacemide and trimethodione, which have now understandably been deleted from the active antiepileptic pharmacopoeia. Even now, in spite of further significant advances in treatment, notably the introduction of carbamazepine and valproate, phenobarbitone is the most widely prescribed medication worldwide for the treatment of epilepsy. It is perhaps the most potent of all the anticonvulsant drugs, is relatively safe, and importantly for many areas of the globe, cheap. Phenobarbitone is no longer a first line drug alongside phenytoin, carbamazepine and valproate, but it still has a place. Its fall from favour is on account of the sedative effect with chronic administration. Toxic manifestations of major consequence, hepatic and haematological, do occur, but are rarer than with some of the more recently introduced compounds.

Phenobarbitone, however, is regarded, and rightly so, as hazardous because of dependency, use as an illicit drug, and importantly because suicidal overdose is extremely dangerous. The long half-life, and therefore extended period of sedation with consequent mortality and morbidity, is a matter of great concern in patients who attempt to take their own life in this way.

Another reason for its relegation to second place, and the label of 'old-fashioned', has been the apparition of the slow, slurred, unsteady, chronic patient who is receiving large doses of phenobarbitone. Often we find that large doses of other antiepileptics are also being given. These might equally be responsible for the intoxicated state. This could be avoided if treatment was with only one drug. The current slogan 'use monotherapy' in management is important, and can be achieved in many patients. Obtaining this state, in those receiving many drugs, reveals another snag of phenobarbitone: it has to be withdrawn extremely slowly, otherwise convulsions are almost inevitable. Withdrawal also has to take place with particular care in those patients who are seizure-free for long periods, and in whom antiepileptic drugs are to be discontinued completely. Even stopping the final 15 milligrams of phenobarbitone may precipitate seizures again.

There are other considerations in relation to this compound. These concern children, the middle-aged and the elderly. In children where this drug is being used as a prophylactic measure to prevent repeated febrile convulsions or for the treatment of a continuing seizure disorder, hyperactivity can be a problem, whereas in the middle-aged and elderly, depressive symptoms are not uncommon, and the drug has to be withdrawn.

CONCLUSION

It appears that the discovery of the antiepileptic effect of phenobarbitone was serendipitous. It could not have happened unless the compound had been synthesized, therefore the observations of Hauptmann occurred against a background of an active chemical industry in Germany. Yet it was Hauptmann's observation that, when used as a sedative in overactive and excited patients with epilepsy, their seizures were controlled, a finding he was to elaborate in various ways and so have enough evidence to publish. Also of interest is the uncertainty that remains about the exact mode of action of phenobarbitone. Finally, it is of note that no one country has contributed all the advances in the drug treatment of epilepsy (see Chapter 1). The efficacy of bromides emerged from England, although interestingly, Locock's observations were based on those of an unknown German. The next major advance, namely phenytoin, was from the US, and other later drugs dealt with in subsequent chapters have other geographical assignations.

REFERENCES

1. Mavromatis, A. (1991). *Hypnagogia: the Unique State of Consciousness Between Wakefulness and Sleep.* (London: Routledge)
2. Ivanov, A. (1964). Soviet experiments in 'eyeless vision'. *Int. J. Parapsychol.*, **6**, 7
3. Hauptmann, A. (1912). Luminal bei epilepsie. *Munch. Med. Wochenschr.*, **59**, 1907
4. Coatsworth, J.J. (1971). Studies on the clinical efficacy of marketed antiepileptic drugs. In NINDS Monograph, No. 12. (Bethesda, Maryland: US Dept. Health Education and Welfare)

5

Epilepsy in the 1930s –
the pre-phenytoin era

At this point we must pause and consider what treatment was available for the patient with epilepsy in the 1930s before the introduction of phenytoin. In addition we must review some of the advances in investigation that were eventually to change radically the overall management of seizure disorders.

It is possible to glimpse at the situation of a patient of this time by the later reminiscences of Dr Tracy Putnam[1]. Though actually a neurosurgeon by training he became very interested in epilepsy. He emphasizes that the standard work of that time was Osler's textbook of medicine, yet it devoted only a few pages to epilepsy and comments were 'lifted' almost verbatim from Hippocrates. Putnam recalls the fate of two relatives, one had pustules on his nose due to bromide and the other was 'shut off from the world' because of epilepsy.

Ignorance and misunderstanding of patients with epilepsy were remnants of earlier ages in history but were to persist for many more years. One patient, Putnam recalls, had half her colon removed in an effort to relieve her seizures, no doubt to improve the surgeon's bank balance rather than to benefit the patient herself!

At this time there were two drug groups available, bromides and barbituric acid derivatives, notably phenobarbitone. The direct surgical treatment of epilepsy was by excision of cortical scars. This method was well-known but rarely carried out, though the first operation had in fact been successfully performed by Sir Victor Horsley on a patient of Dr Hughlings Jackson (see Chapter 7). Indeed Osler's textbook recalls, according to Putnam, 30 different types of operation, not necessarily on the head, reported to alleviate seizures. There was another treatment available at this time, the ketogenic diet. This was not only important in itself but fostered the understanding that epilepsy was a biochemical disorder. Also becoming widely appreciated at this time was the fact that many patients with epilepsy did not have any structural abnormality as the cause of their seizures. Electroencephalography, though in its infancy, helped to introduce the notion of seizures being a disordered pattern of the brain's electrical activity. Technological advance has been important for progress in the treatment of epilepsy, as shown by the introduction of X-ray techniques such as angiography which came about towards the end of the third decade and had an important impact on management.

THE KETOGENIC DIET

It had been observed much earlier by physicians at the time of Hippocrates and even before this, that fasting could result in control of epilepsy. Biblical references, too, indicated that prayer and fasting were important therapies. It was Geyelin in 1921 who began a resurgence of interest in diet with a more organized approach to this matter[2]. A year later Conklin also reported success[3], and about this time Wilder made the suggestion that it was probably the ketone bodies, produced by starvation, that were anticonvulsant[4]. He produced at the Mayo Clinic a diet which would produce ketosis but provide, in addition, sufficient calories and other requirements to maintain a satisfactory nutritional state and not inhibit the growth rate, because this treatment was often used for children with petit mal. This was the main problem, to give enough calories and other dietary factors not only to allow for day-to-day activities but also sufficient for normal growth and development. It was Woodyatt who published such a diet and staff at the Mayo Clinic used the detailed instructions for many years, even as recently as in the 1960s[5]. This mainly involved eating large quantities of fat whilst restricting both protein and carbohydrate intake. The excretion of ketones in the urine, which could easily be assessed, acted as a check of progress.

Such a regime is not well tolerated when started abruptly, but the aim was to introduce it gradually over 4–6 days and then, remarkably, the diet seemed to be acceptable without the nausea and vomiting which one might have predicted. To be effective it had to be carefully controlled and this involved weighing foods and the frequent checking of urine samples, as well as careful attention to weight.

The diet is primarily intended to control seizures in children, so clearly the mother was an important figure and constant help and instruction by a dietician was essential.

Using the ketogenic method it was possible to control seizures. The effect occurred in some patients in a few days but in others the diet might be needed to be continued for weeks to check efficacy. Clearly this would reinforce the importance of maintaining the diet. Generally a trial for 3 months was worthwhile and if there was no success by then the method was discontinued. Using the various details to establish the exact constituents for the particular weight of the child required a fairly complex formula but even then hunger was a problem. Not unexpectedly, in view of the high fat intake, nausea and vomiting were often prominent features.

As with any diet there were problems at home because one member of the family required special attention. The diet which had to be prepared separately from the other family food was time-consuming, also young children tended to succumb to the temptations of 'forbidden' items. It was also quite clear to schoolmates that this child was having a particular, and indeed peculiar diet, and could not, as the others did, eat sweets, chew gum, or have popular highly sugar-containing drinks.

The ketogenic diet could be administered with antiepileptic drugs and reduction of sedative phenobarbitone was possible. It is not surprising that trials of this method showed that quite a proportion of patients for various reasons could not adhere to the strict regimen, but of those that did, whatever type of seizure they had, a third were virtually fit-free. At this time only phenobarbitone and bromides were available. Clearly the response was remarkable. Keith quotes results of various studies, not only from America, but also from Europe, which indicated the beneficial effect[5]. Livingstone, in 1954, was an advocate of the system[6], and he had treated more than 300 patients and reported control of attacks in a remarkable 44%. It was most effective in the 2–5 year olds. Keith reports not only the overall findings, but cites individual case histories and shows remarkable improvement in EEG features when a ketogenic diet is used.

Clearly this dieting approach was superseded by the introduction in the 1940s and 1950s of other drugs, in particular tridione, and the succinamides. They were, with much less effort, able to control the petit mal attacks which were markedly responsive to a ketogenic diet.

ACETAZOLAMIDE

So often the rationale for the introduction of a compound into therapy proves to be invalid yet the treatment actually works! This was the case with acetazolamide (Diamox®), a carbonic anhydrase inhibitor. Its use was considered as a substitute for the acidosis-producing ketogenic diet. The first hint that such a compound might be effective came in the late 1930s when sulphonamides were introduced for the treatment of infection[7]. They had the effect of reducing carbonic anhydrase in the brain, and thereby producing acidosis, considered to be the mechanism for antiepileptic action.

However, this was not followed up until much later with the introduction of acetazolamide, as an adjunctive treatment[8]. This drug's action in patients, like that of many other medications, tends to 'wear off' with the passage of time, that is, tolerance is developed. As a result, the drug came to be used less and less. Then suddenly, almost like a fashion in the clothing trade, it re-appeared in 1989, shown in a detailed clinical trial to be an effective 'helper' drug. This was particularly the case in the most resistant type of epilepsy in which complex partial seizures were a notable feature[9]. About half the patients showed a good response without toxic effect.

THE DISCOVERY OF ELECTROENCEPHALOGRAPHY

Advances in the treatment of epilepsy were, and still are, not entirely related to drug treatment. It is trite to observe that accurate diagnosis not only precedes proper management but also aids in prognosis. One technique, electroencephalography (EEG), in spite of certain limitations was, and still is, of great importance. EEG started from very humble beginnings in Germany in a psychiatric institution. The year of the first publication, by Hans Berger, was 1929 and though it was in German and is a relatively little-known journal[10,11], by the early 1930s there were exponents of the technique both in Europe, the UK and the USA. This is remarkable, especially bearing in mind the technical problems, for at that time electronics had not been developed as a specialty. Perhaps also surprising is the fact that recording of electrical impulses from the human head had not been reported before, because studies of the electrical activity of the nervous system

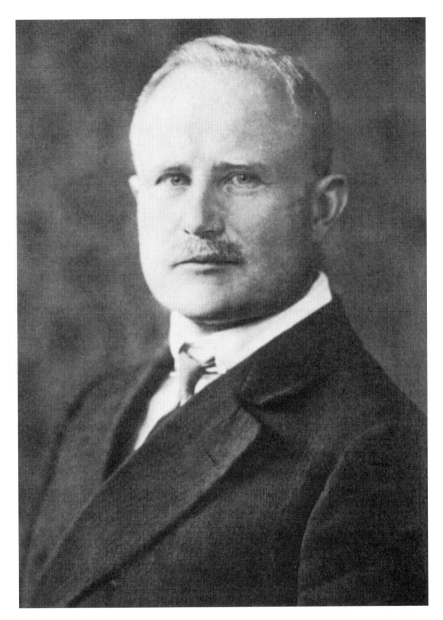

Figure 1 Hans Berger in 1925, aged 52, one year after beginning work on the human electroencephalogram. (Reproduced by kind permission of the publishers, Elsevier Science, and the author, Pierre Gloor, from 'Hans Berger on the Electroencephalogram of Man'[11])

in various animals had been carried out. In the UK as early as 1869 Caton demonstrated to a British Medical Association meeting just such an observation.

Yet others were highly sceptical of Berger's reports – they probably did not in the first instance believe that it was possible to record anything of significance from the surface of the brain through the scalp muscles. Jasper[12] later stated the difficulty in view of 'the enormous complexity of action potentials which must be coursing in all directions in the multitude of nerve cells and fibres of the brain', yet indeed it was not only possible, but achievable as Berger showed.

His first paper published in 1929[10] described simple rhythmic waves which he designated the 'alpha-und-beta Wellen'. Others asked could they really represent something that was genuine and important?

Jasper described his visit to Jena (Figure 2) where Berger worked as follows: 'this was an unforgettable experience to be cherished for many years to come, for I was profoundly impressed by this inspired and inspiring, humble, honest, friendly, distinguished and courageous man'. This visit was at the time the Nazis were beginning to present a danger.

In fact Berger had begun his work on neurophysiology before the First World War and had persisted in spite of technical difficulties and the criticism of sceptical colleagues. Subsequently he made use of the many patients with skull defects that resulted from the First World War, proving that electrical waves could be recorded and were truly representative of electrical activity of the brain beneath.

The discovery of the electroencephalogram by Berger was clearly not a chance phenomenon. It exemplifies the comment of Thomas Edison the American scientist, 'genius is one per cent inspiration and 99 per cent perspiration'. Berger's aim, which is now only being in part realized, was to link mental disease to the electroencephalogram. As Jasper states, 'he was convinced that careful investigation of the workings of the brain, by objective scientific methods, would lead eventually to the understanding of disease itself, its normal functions in sleeping and waking, and its derangement in a mental disease'.

Just how extensive was Berger's hard work is exemplified by the fact that he published 102 papers and monographs during his scientific career. Twenty-eight of these 102 publications dealt with the EEG. Almost all were written in German.

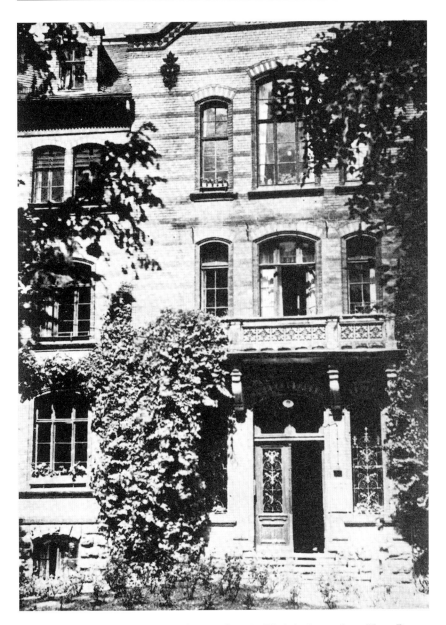

Figure 2   The main entrance to the Psychiatric Clinic in Jena where Hans Berger worked. The window on the left of doorway belongs to the room where Berger's recordings were performed[11]. (Reproduced by kind permission of Elsevier Science and Pierre Gloor)

BERGER'S PRE-1914 STUDIES

Berger's first ever paper was published in 1898 on 'the generation of the anterior horn cells of the spinal cord in dementia paralytica'. He continued with some animal studies and became particularly interested in blood flow in the cranial cavity and how it could be changed by various drugs. He carried out tracings from a patient with a pulsating skull defect and developed the cerebral plethysmograph. His early published recordings from 1929 onwards show such tracings in addition to the EEG. He was familiar with the experimental animal work carried out by Caton and other Europeans. By 1902 he was attempting to record the electrical activity of the cerebral cortex of a dog, and he continued these studies with the use of a string galvanometer. His diaries record progress or often lack of it. Yet in 1910 after the failure to obtain potentials from the cerebral cortex of dogs, he was not dissuaded from continuing.

During these years Berger measured temperature changes in the cerebral cortex and response to various stimuli. His work was interrupted by the 1914–18 War, but at the end of it he returned to the University of Jena and was appointed to the Chair of Psychiatry. Quite quickly he began further attempts to record electrical activity of the human brain through the scalp. His first unsuccessful attempt was in 1920 using a 'bald medical student'. He continued stimulation experiments and, as Gloor states, in a diary entry of 1924 there was clearly the beginning of his ultimate success – 'the idea to search for cortical potentials in humans with palliative trephenations'.

BERGER'S TECHNIQUE

Berger was ill-prepared for recording the human electroencephalogram because of his limited knowledge of physics and instrumentation. He relied on apparatus which used an optical recording system. A beam of light deflected from the moving mirror was recorded on photographic paper (Figure 3). The lengths of the record obtained varied from 2.5 to 7.5 metres. He did not have the luxury which we now have of multichannel apparatus, although he clearly had hoped that such a system would become available. He tried a variety of electrodes, eventually employing the needle inserted into the skin, still used now

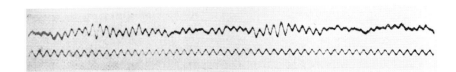

Figure 3 Recording from Klaus, Berger's son, at the age of 15 years. A double-coil galvanometer was used; the electrodes were placed on the forehead and the occiput. The upper tracing is an EEG, the lower is a time calibration signal with 10 waves per second[10,11]. (Reproduced by kind permission of Elsevier Science and Pierre Gloor)

for certain purposes. These were placed near to the skull defect which resulted either from neurosurgical procedures or following cranial injury. For those without skull defect, electrodes were held in place with a band, and usually situated one in the frontal and the other in the occipital region.

It is therefore quite clear that Berger's discoveries were the result of genius coupled with '99 per cent perspiration'. He succeeded in spite of repeated disappointments and many difficulties. As Gloor[11] comments: '... one can only marvel at the determination and single-mindedness with which Berger pursued his goal, for most of the early tracings show little more than a straight line with only a very occasional deflection, which can hardly be interpreted as convincing evidence of cerebral activity'. Many might have given up the struggle at that stage but he, in spite of discouragement and despair as reported in his detailed personal diary, convinced himself of the reality of the observations he had made. It was then that he had to persuade others that what he had seen on his tracings was in fact electrical activity from the brain, and not artefacts generated by the apparatus, or extraneous potentials resulting from non-cortical structures. Even as late as a year before his first paper on the subject, Berger was almost ready to abandon his studies!

The investigations were always carried out at the end of the day's work at the Clinic, between five and eight pm when there was less electrical interference. Also to help in this respect, the electrical supply in the building where he worked and those adjacent, was turned off. In fact even today in many situations when there is much electrical equipment attached to the patient, for example in the Intensive Therapy Unit, mains interference can prove a real problem!

Berger's first paper had little impact. He remained lonely and isolated. The resistance to acceptance of his findings was partly from those who were expert neurophysiologists, which he was not. They were familiar with spiky action potentials and were sceptical of the regular undulations he demonstrated from the brain, particularly because these could be recorded through the intact skull, thus adding to their general doubt. Another reason for doubting Berger's findings was his personality. He was shy and reticent, finding social intercourse difficult, though his diary shows that he was an extraordinary person with considerable communication skills. His rigid timetable of work, his strict and meticulous manner made everyone regard him as unimaginative. He was recognized as an excellent neurologist who was able clinically to localize lesions, though never applying the EEG to this end, yet it was in this respect, following the report published by Walter[13] in *The Lancet* in 1936, that the subject gained kudos. For Berger, as for so many innovators, it was his closest colleagues who were unaware of his discovery and were blind to his absorbing scientific aspirations.

The political background in Germany of the rise of the Nazis also disrupted Berger's work and it was finally to be instrumental in his death. He was deposed in 1938 from his post and lived through an unhappy retirement for a further 3 years, until in the depths of a severe depressive illness he committed suicide.

The high point of Berger's career was his attendance at the International Congress of Psychology in Paris in 1938, where he found, apparently to his own surprise, that he was an international celebrity, the father of electroencephalography. By this time neurophysiologists in France, Belgium, Germany and the United States were already thoroughly involved in electroencephalography and the distinguished neurophysiologists, Adrian and Matthews[14], had in fact suggested that the alpha rhythm be known as the 'Berger rhythm', but apparently Berger himself was not keen on this idea, and the terminology quickly reverted to the 'alpha rhythm' as he had originally suggested.

BERGER'S IDEAS AND ENERGY

No-one could doubt Berger's meticulousness, after reading his first paper[10], more recently available in an excellent translation[11]. The first communication traces his long and arduous path to the conviction that the lines on the photographic paper indicated potentials from the brain. Once again we can be impressed by the amount and duration of methodical work which has to be coupled with the imaginative idea in order to convey it to the world in a form that is acceptable. Everything was against him. He lacked technical background, so it seemed unlikely that a psychiatrist working in isolation could make such an original observation as well as discover and sustain his findings against so many odds, not forgetting the unstable political background against which he worked.

His first paper demonstrated that regular oscillations could be recorded from skull defects and from the scalp of the intact skull. He showed in a carefully designed series of experiments that these oscillations could not be accounted for by pulsations caused by blood flow through the cerebral vessels or through the scalp vessels, nor could they be attributed to cranial musculature, eye movements or the psychogalvanic potentials arising directly from the skin. Berger also showed that these oscillations could not be due to the electro-cardiogram. In addition he demonstrated that the pulse wave in the scalp vessels bore no relationship to the regular oscillations of the electroencephalogram. He later showed in a subsequent paper from a patient undergoing a diagnostic procedure, that these potentials could be recorded directly from the cerebral cortex itself and were not arising from the white matter.

The real interest in these observations to him was the relationship of what he had recorded to psychological processes. Berger quickly observed that the oscillations – the alpha waves – disappeared with eye opening and that other forms of stimulation, such as touch, noise and pain, as well as intellectual activity such as performing mental arithmetic, had similar effects. The oscillations – alpha waves – disappear when the subject is alerted. This, of course, was in contrast to animal work by many neurophysiologists showing that stimulation indeed produced increases in the recorded electrical activity from the skull. He also noted that alpha waves were not seen in the immature brain of the newborn, or in the adult during chloroform anaesthesia and in postictal coma. However, the observation he made that patients with manic depressive illness and schizophrenia, as well as those with mental retardation, showed normal records, was a profound disappointment.

Berger and mental activities

On the basis of his observations Berger built up various theories of mental activity as well as of the origin of the alpha rhythm. For example, he gained the impression, as Gloor[11] indicates, that 'the synchronization of the electrical oscillations generated by the two cerebral hemispheres', reflected in uniform waves of activity in the EEG, spread 'in a sagittal direction over both hemispheres'. He assumed that this cortical activity was regulated by a thalamic centre which also kept the activity of cerebral neurons within certain bounds.

This, and many other concepts, such as 'inhibition' and the problems of 'signal-to-noise ratio' are still important to our understanding, as is his view that structural changes can occur in the nervous system as a basis for the learning process.

Berger and epilepsy

Over the 10 years or more in which Berger worked in this field he recorded the EEG in a great number of different pathological states. He was aware that slow waves in the EEG were associated with many kinds of cerebral lesion. He also knew, for example, that in vascular lesions the EEG became 'inactive' but could revert to normal. He made many interesting observations on epilepsy (Figure 4). Indeed it is truly remarkable that he described phenomena in many types of epilepsy. His one disappointment was never to obtain a satisfactory recording from a generalized tonic/clonic seizure, but he gave credit to Gibbs, Lennox and Gibbs[16] for just such an observation. However, even now we are well aware that there are real problems with recordings during seizures because of the often overwhelming muscle and movement artefact.

Berger did record minor seizures with loss of consciousness and these were almost certainly varieties of temporal lobe epilepsy, which we would now call simple or complex partial fits. He noted that following attacks there was a postictal depression of cerebral activity which could be profound. He also observed high-voltage, three cycles per second, wave patterns in 'absence' attacks – classically petit mal seizures. His tracings did not show the spike component, and he took several years to decide whether to publish these observations,

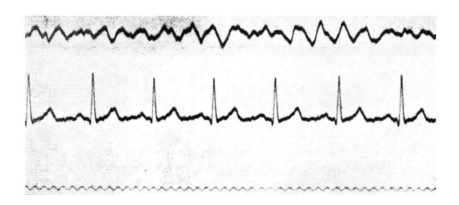

Figure 4 Recording from a 35-year-old woman with epilepsy. The upper tracing is an EEG showing a jagged pattern from needle electrodes placed over the left frontal and right occipital regions. The middle tracing is an ECG, and the lower a time calibration with waves at 10 per second[11,15]. (Reproduced by kind permission of Elsevier Science and Pierre Gloor)

because he regarded the high voltage oscillations as probably artefactual in type. His American contemporaries published an EEG, showing the spike and wave pattern, at about the same time (Figure 5).

Berger, however, was well aware that high-voltage waves which appeared suddenly were characteristic of the EEG of epileptic patients between seizures. This was published in the seventh report, his most valuable contribution to the EEG in epilepsy. It concerned a patient who had general paralysis of the insane and focal motor seizures. He demonstrated that discharges were localized to the left central region, approximately over the motor area, and these preceded the observed movements, which were localized jerks. Berger monitored these by means of a pulse telephone which was put on the patient's hand.

This striking finding was the first directly to prove the correctness of Hughlings Jackson's hypothesis, that excessive discharges in the grey matter related to a clinical seizure, the electrical manifestation of the attack at a particular site producing the appropriate clinical phenomena. Yet Berger seems to have been unaware of Jackson's work which could have furnished him with even greater fervour, since both Jackson's views on seizures and also the hierarchical arrangement of the nervous system would obviously have appealed.

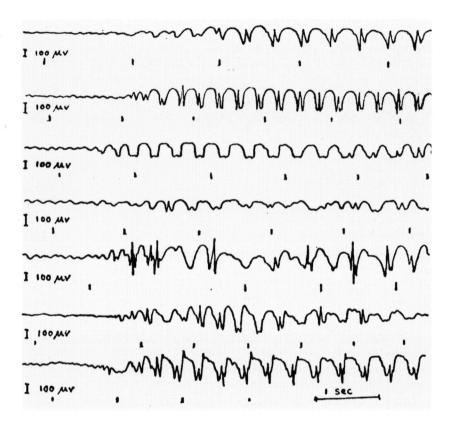

Figure 5 One of the first published EEGs, showing the spike and wave, or spike and dome, pattern occurring three times per second, characteristic of petit mal seizures (seen most clearly on the second line from the top of the tracing). The dots are the time marker indicating seconds[17]. (Reproduced by kind permission)

Berger amply demonstrates one who grasped a particular concept, would not let it go and found supportive evidence eventually, in spite of overwhelming difficulty. In his case the observations seemed not to be the result of chance or luck but simply hard work. In the words of the philosopher, Francis Bacon (1561–1626) 'a wise man will make more opportunities than he finds'. Berger had to prove to a sceptical and hostile world that his findings were not only correct, but of value. That they were has been shown by the advances in the field still continuing more than 60 years later. He would almost certainly have greatly appreciated that there were potentials recordable which relate directly to mental processing[18]. Now elegant techniques exist for stimulating the brain magnetically to produce changes at the periphery as well as the reverse. Also complex electrodes can now be used both on the surface and in the deep structures of the brain. These have led to progress in epilepsy surgery, a field at present rapidly advancing (see Chapter 12).

NEURORADIOLOGY

The history of radiology, and in particular neuroradiology, proceeded in parallel with the discovery of EEG, first in animals and then in man. Caton's demonstration of electrical activity from animals was followed by the discovery of X-rays by Röntgen (1845–1923), at Würzburg in Germany, whose first report was in 1895. Neuro-radiology was fathered by Arthur Schüller who qualified a year after Röntgen's original publication. Surprisingly Schüller was trained in neurophysiology and yet in his radiological practice he was never interested in contrast methods, skull X-rays being his forte. They of course do not demonstrate any significant detail of the brain itself.

The first 'contrast' pictures in radiology which show the brain occurred by chance. The patient with skull fractures extending through the frontal sinuses allowed the entry of air into the cranial cavity. Such spontaneous pneumoencephalography stimulated the neurosurgeon Dandy to introduce air to the lumbar theca, after removal of an equivalent amount of cerebrospinal fluid with the patient in a sitting position, and to take radiographs of the head. Dandy also introduced the technique of ventriculography and the discussion of this at a meeting was reported in the journal *Brain*. It was read subsequently by Moniz, the Professor of Medicine, in Lisbon. He, not satisfied with ventriculography, was spurred on to another method of investigation which led to the discovery of cerebral angiography, a major step forward[19]. In particular Moniz was impressed by the work of Sicard who had introduced a positive contrast substance to outline the spinal theca.

Moniz observed that the brain was normally mute to X-rays, being a 'dark continent'. He chose for his contrast a medium containing an aqueous solution of an iodine salt. After animal experimentation sodium iodide was selected. The first attempt at this technique was unsuccessful, but after study of cadavers he enlisted the help of his pupil and successor, Lima, to carry out the injections. This percutaneous method again proved unsuccessful but Moniz was not deterred. He suggested that the medium had not entered the artery, and from then on he decided to expose the vessel surgically, to ensure that the substance was definitely in the circulatory system.

His tremendous determination was rewarded in 1927 when he read a paper about the results in Paris[20]. Four years later a monograph on the subject described the findings in his first 90 patients[21]. The preface was written by none other than the famous neurologist, Babinski, who praised his enterprise in charting the 'dark continent'.

The technique of demonstrating the cerebral ventricles was improved by Lysholm working in Stockholm. He showed by 1937 that supratentorial space-occupying masses, such as tumours, could be readily demonstrated. The technique of angiography was also improved by taking additional films from different directions, not only anterior and posterior but also lateral projections, with rapid serial X-rays, which could show how contrast filled the arterial side of the circulation as well as filling, moments later, the sinuses and veins.

The next advance in imaging was presented by Moore, a surgeon from the USA, in 1948. He invented the technique of the isotope brain scan. It depends on the observation that, for example, rapidly growing tumours assimilate radioactive isotopes which, because they give out radiation, are detected on X-ray films. This avoided the possibility of morbidity and discomfort experienced in angiography, though by this time is was routinely percutaneous and the artery did not need to be exposed surgically. The cut-down technique of Moniz had been abandoned by most radiologists. Though the isotope brain scan in now rarely used, the technique is still applied for the detection of disseminated cancerous lesions, particularly in the bones.

COMPUTERIZED TOMOGRAPHY

The next leap forward, which was indeed a real high jump, came from Jeffrey Hounsfield who first published in 1973[22] an account of his invention termed computerized tomography. This was rewarded with a Nobel Prize only a very few years later, in 1979. It is without doubt the greatest advance in radiology since Röntgen's original discovery of X-rays[19]. Although it was possible to examine all systems of the body with this technique, the investigation of the nervous system, in particular of the brain, benefited most initially.

Hounsfield's advances arose from pattern recognition studies at the EMI company in Middlesex, England. Basically X-ray 'slices' were taken and from these, by a computerized technique, it was possible to produce a three-dimensional representation of the soft tissue structures, which were not distinguishable by conventional X-ray methods. The other necessary advance was the replacement of photographic plates by a matrix of crystals which scintillated when exposed to X-rays. This allowed a much greater resolution of detail than was possible using traditional photographic methods. Computers were essential to process the data, that could then be demonstrated as the usual type of X-ray film, with which the radiologist was familiar. Initially the technique was slow and required hours to perform but later the time factor was greatly reduced, first to minutes and then to fractions of a second.

This was all very much in the future and we must return to the 1930s and to the next advance in drug treatment.

REFERENCES

1. Putnam, T.J. (1970). Demonstration of specific anticonvulsant action of diphenylhydantoin and related compounds. In Ayd, F.J. Jr. (ed.) *Discoveries in Biological Psychiatry Symposium, Baltimore.* Ayd Medical Communications, 85
2. Geyelin, H.R. (1921). Fasting as a method for treating epilepsy. *Med. Record*, **99**, 1037
3. Conklin, H.W. (1922). Cause and treatment of epilepsy. *J. Am. Osteopathol. Assoc.*, **22**, 11
4. Wilder, R.M. (1921). The effect of ketonemia on the course of epilepsy. *Mayo Clinic Bull.*, **2**, 307
5. Keith, Haddow, M. (1963). *Convulsive Disorders in Children with Reference to the Treatment with Ketogenic Diet.* (London: Churchill)
6. Livingstone, S. (1954). *The Diagnosis and Treatment of Convulsive Disorders in Children.* (Springfield, Illinois: Charles C. Thomas)
7. Yeoman, J.C. (1938). Sulphonamide in epilepsy. *Br. Med. J.*, **2**, 261
8. Ansell, B. and Clarke, E. (1956). Epilepsy and menstruation. *Lancet*, **2**, 1232

9.   Oles, K.S., Penry, J.K., Cole, D.L.W. and Howard, G. (1989). Use of acetozolamide as an adjunct to carbamazepine in refractory partial seizures. *Epilepsia*, **30**, 74

10. Berger, H. (1929). On the electroencephalogram of man. First Report. *Archiv für Psychiatrik und Nervenkrankheiter*, **87**, 527

11. Gloor, P. (Translator) (1969). Hans Berger on the electroencephalogram of man: the fourteen original reports on the human electroencephalogram. *Electroencephalogr. Clin. Neurophysiol.*, (Suppl. 28)

12. Jasper, H.H. (1969). Preface in Gloor, P. Hans Berger on the electroencephalogram of man. *Electroencephalogr. Clin. Neurphysiol.*, (Suppl. 28). (See also refs 10, 11)

13. Walter, W.G. (1936). Location of cerebral tumours by electroencephalography. *Lancet*, **2**, 305

14. Adrian, E.D. and Matthews, B.H.C. (1934). The Berger rhythm. Potential changes from the occipital lobes in man. *Brain*, **57**, 355

15. Berger, H. (1931). On the electroencephalogram of man. Third report. *Archiv für Psychiatrik und Nervenkrankheiter*, **94**, 16. (See also ref. 11)

16. Gibbs, F.A., Lennox, W. and Gibbs, E. (1936). The electroencephalogram during seizures. *Arch. Neurol. Psychiatry*, **36**, 1225

17. Gibbs, F.A., Davis, H. and Lennox, W.G. (1935). The electroencephalogram during petit mal. *Arch. Neurol. Psychiatry*, **34**, 193

18. Walter, W.G., Cooper, R., Aldridge, J., McCallum, W.C. and Winter, A.L. (1964). Contingent negative variation: An electric sign of sensorimotor association and expectancy in the human brain. *Nature (London)*, **203**, 380

19. Bull, N. (1982). History of neuroradiology. In Rose, C.F. and Bynam, M. (eds.) *History of the Neurosciences*. (New York: Raven)

20. Moniz, E. (1927). Cerebral angiography. *Rev. Neurol.*, **34**, ii, 72

21. Moniz, E. (1931). *Diagnostic des tumeurs cérebrales et épreuve l'encephalographie artérielles*. (Paris: Masson)

22. Hounsfield, J.N. (1973). Computerised transverse axial scanning (Tomography). Part I. Description of system. *Br. J. Radiol.*, **46**, 1016

6

Phenytoin – a major advance

In the history of the discovery of anticonvulsants, the combination of chance, luck and serendipity could not better be illustrated than with the discovery of phenytoin by Putnam. It is also interesting that the full report of this breakthrough in the treatment of epilepsy did not appear until 50 years after the event[1]. Credit for this advance must also be given to the part played by the drug firm, Parke Davis, and its staff. In relation to other drugs, different companies have been important, and as we noted, perhaps remarkably, the discoveries have been made in several different countries. It has already been seen that the benefit of bromides was reported first in England and phenobarbitone in Germany. With phenytoin the US takes the laurels. The compound was first synthesized by Biltz in 1908, and as with others there is a considerable latency, here of 30 years, before it reached the pharmacy shelves.

The story of the establishment of phenytoin as a major antiepileptic drug has many facets. First of all there is the question of animal models. There has been much discussion of the ethics of animal experimentation recently (see Chapter 12), but it is clear that the development of a method of screening, in this case using the cat, was a crucial step, almost as important as the chemical itself. Putnam and his colleagues were responsible for this on the basis of previous work[2], but it was Putnam's singular grasp of organic chemistry, in particular molecular structure in relation to drug action, and his ability to track down the substances he suspected might be effective, that was all-important. The role of his clinical colleague, Merritt, was extremely valuable, indeed some believe that his contribution to this advance in therapy has never received its proper acknowledgement. He was also involved in some of the animal experimentation[1].

An indication of their joint industry is shown by the large number of chemicals examined. Out of the 746 eventually tested, 76 compounds were found to raise the convulsive threshold for the cat without problems of toxicity. The list included not only many substances in the hydantoin series, but also diones which were a series of compounds to prove particularly useful in petit mal epilepsy[3].

They then carried out clinical trials on patients resistant to phenytoin, with the substances which were found in the cat model to be effective. In addition, they began chronic toxicity trials in animals, with a view to their use of other compounds in human studies.

THE ANIMAL MODEL

The equipment used (Figure 1) was crude by modern standards, but was able to produce a standard shock, so for each animal there was a characteristic threshold which did not vary by more than 10% from day to day. The cat was placed in the restraining box and a shaven area of skin between the ears was used for the placement of an electrode. The other electrode was placed in the mouth. The current was turned on for 10 seconds.

Early studies by Putnam and Merritt in 1937[4] showed that, though bromide, in a dose that prevented the cat from walking, raised the threshold by 50%, a dose of phenobarbitone high enough to produce the same behavioural effect raised the convulsive threshold by three or four times. However, phenytoin showed a dissociation between antiepileptic and toxic effects which was more striking.

Even after the finding of phenytoin, work continued in a search for other substances which might be more successful. Their animal model was shown to produce repeatable results, so they were able to test the effect of various compounds in raising the seizure threshold, and obtain an index of efficacy of any substance under study. The current, measured in milliamps, was applied for 10 seconds and repeated after 5 minutes[3]. They observed that, 'by this method a convulsive seizure can be produced with regularity'. A baseline value was obtained and the compound administered. Then the test was repeated after 2–3 hours time to allow for drug absorption. This was generally given in liquid form by mouth. Antiepileptic compounds, such as phenobarbitone and phenytoin, would raise the baseline

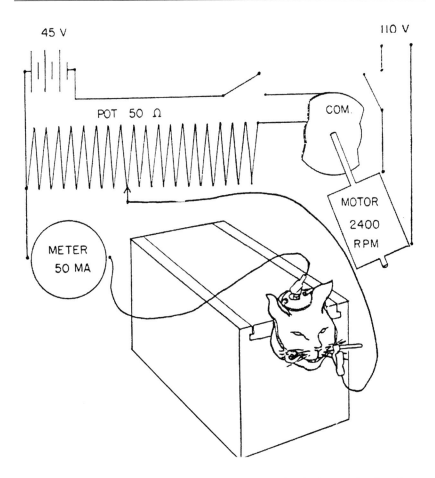

Figure 1 The circuit Putnam and Merritt employed, which permitted an interrupted current of predetermined amperage to be applied through the animal's head, to obtain the threshold for convulsions[4]. (Copyright 1937 by American Association for the Advancement of Science. Reproduced with permission)

level of 10–15 milliamps to 50 or more milliamps. Several tests were made with each substance with increasing dosage until toxic symptoms appeared.

In this way, Merritt and Putnam were able not only to list substances that elevated the convulsive threshold, but also to obtain signs of untoward effects, such as inability to walk steadily, or with more severe toxicity, for example, inability of the animals to stand or walk. The studies were very extensive and the results from the 746 compounds were presented in tabular form in 1945[3], just 8 years after the method had been proven.

STRUCTURE AND ACTIVITY RELATIONSHIPS

The next part of the jigsaw concerned the chemicals to be screened for antiepileptic activity. Because bromides were sedative, the relationship between sedation and antiepileptic effects was appreciated. This had been the pathway to the use of phenobarbitone.

It was natural that chemists would substitute other molecular groups to obtain compounds in the barbiturate series which might be successful hypnotics. Dox and Thomas, two organic chemists working in the Parke Davis laboratories in 1923, prepared phenyl derivatives of barbituric acid[1]. These were not notable in their hypnotic effect, but they also mentioned that hydantoins had a ring structure which was similar to the barbiturates, and in particular they noted that diphenylhydantoin with two phenyl rings was totally devoid of hypnotic action, and so of little interest as a marketable pharmaceutical compound at that stage. As Glazko[1] reported:

'This may explain why 5,5,diphenylhydantoin was sitting on the shelf in a Parke Davis laboratory, just waiting to be discovered as an anticonvulsive drug, a whole decade later!'

PUTNAM'S MAJOR CONTRIBUTION

Once the screening test for antiepileptic action in animals was fully developed, Putnam was in a position to test a variety of compounds for their efficacy in this respect. Apart from this, his major contribution was to separate the hypnotic and antiepileptic action of drugs (Figure 2). He did not assume, as had previously been the case, that a good hypnotic was of necessity an effective antiepileptic. He related such an action to the presence of a phenyl ring in the molecule, and began to search for compounds related to phenobarbitone, but with this additional group. Putnam[5] writes much later about his findings:

'I combed the Eastman Chemical Company's catalogue, and other price lists, for suitable phenyl compounds that were not

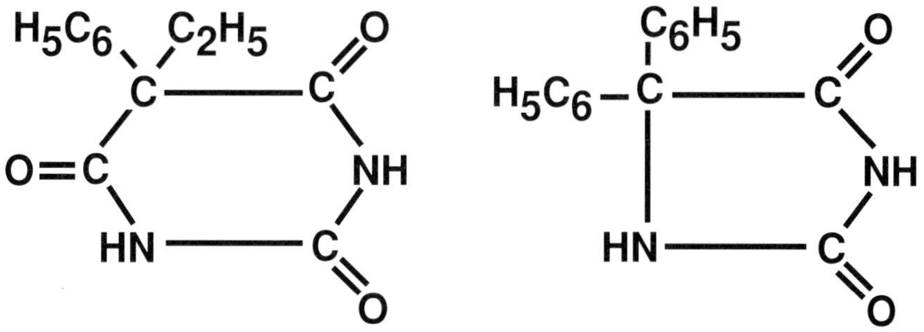

Figure 2 Chemical formulae of phenobarbitone on the left and phenytoin on the right. Note the basic similarity of the molecules, though the ring structure of phenobarbitone has six atoms, while that of phenytoin has only five. Each contains two nitrogen atoms

obviously poisonous. I also wrote to the major pharmaceutical firms, asking if they had available or could make suitable chemicals. The only one of them that showed any interest was Parke, Davis and Company. They wrote back to me that they had on hand samples of 19 different compounds analogous to phenobarbital, and that I was welcome to them.'

The compounds that Putnam was seeking were those that had already been synthesized by Dox, and found to have no hypnotic action. He felt convinced of a relationship between structure and activity, hence his catalogue search and request to Parke Davis. It is of interest that in their files the following note is included[1]:

'To the director of Parke, Davis, a request for compounds to the attention of Dr W. Dox and his new assistant, Dr W. Glen Bywater.'

The Scientific Director of Parke Davis, Dr Kamm, sent a memo on April 3rd, 1936 to Dr Dox and stated,

'In a recent letter, Dr Tracey J. Putnam … expressed an interest in cooperating with us in a search for a barbituric acid hypnotic of the luminal type. He expressed the opinion that certain

---

Compounds sent to Dr. T. J. Putnam from the Parke, Davis laboratories on April 24, 1936

(1) 5,5-diphenylhydantoin
(2) *N*-phenylbarbital
(3) *N*-phenyl-ethylpropylbarbituric acid
(4) *N*-*p*-methoxyphenylbarbital
(5) *N*-*p*-ethoxyphenylbarbital
(6) *N*-benzylbarbital
(7) *N*-*p*-tolylbarbital

From Parke, Davis & Co. research files

Figure 3 List of compounds sent to Dr T.J. Putnam from Parke Davis laboratories on April 24th, 1936. Note that diphenylhydantoin (phenytoin) was the first requested. (From Parke Davis and Co. research files, see Glazko[1])

substances, although rejected as hypnotics, might possess anticonvulsant activity.'

This was the first clear statement of Putnam's view that the two pharmacological properties of antiepileptic activity and hypnotic effect could be separate entities.

Bywater, Dox's assistant, was given the task of selecting from the shelves the drug samples for testing (Figure 3). There were 2 g samples available, and the list in the Parke Davis files shows that of the 19 compounds requested, the first was diphenylhydantoin, phenytoin. Chance had clearly played a card! It seemed conceivable, if this had been the last on the list, that enthusiasm in the screening programme might well have waned before an effective substance on the list was tested. It does appear also at that stage that the experimental model described earlier had not been completely finalized, for Putnam wrote as follows:

'It seems to me that the way to go at it is to devise an experimental set-up which will display the peculiarities of phenobarbital in animals and then apply the same method with this list of drugs.'

This was in a letter of April 15th 1936, and by November 30th of the same year, Dr Putnam wrote to Parke Davis as follows:

'We have at last succeeded in devising a thoroughly satisfactory preparation for testing anticonvulsants in which a cat can be given a convulsion at a surprisingly constant threshold by means of a well-controlled electric current. A dose of phenobarbital too small to cause observable depression will double this threshold in cats. None of the drugs you sent me had a noticeable effect on the convulsive level short of the hypnotic dose except the diphenyl-allantoin which appears to be effective in a smaller dose than luminal. Whether it has a higher therapeutic index remains to be seen, but the results at present are encouraging…'

THE DISCOVERY OF PHENYTOIN

It is thus quite clear that 1936 was the crucial year in the discovery of phenytoin, at that stage known as diphenylhydantoin, and by the middle of the following year, a paper appeared in the journal *Science*, setting out the details of the animal model described above, and also some preliminary results[4]. Later that year some more extensive findings were published[6]. These indicated a dose of the compound that prevented convulsions in the absence of the side-effects shown by phenobarbitone. In particular it did not have any noticeable sedative effect at the dose level employed.

By August 1937, a report was sent to Parke Davis on the treatment of eight patients. Though the length of treatment was only 1–10 weeks, and two of the patients tolerated the drug poorly, it showed a reduction of two-thirds in the number of grand mal attacks. There were two patients with petit mal who showed only marginal benefit.

Quite quickly clinical trials were established, and by September 1938 findings were reported to the Annual Meeting of the American Medical Association, with observations on 200 patients[7]. It was in this year that 'dilantin sodium' was added to the catalogue price list of Parke Davis, but not until the 1950s in Europe, and in 1975 in the US, was the generic name 'phenytoin' adopted.

THE PLACE OF PHENYTOIN IN THE 1990s

Phenytoin still competes with other much more recent antiepileptic compounds such as carbamazepine and sodium valproate, and remains one of the first-line antiepileptic drugs. It controls to a varying extent all types of seizure except petit mal. However, as with other drugs, there is a cost to be paid in side-effects. Indeed, even in the very first group of eight patients reported by Merritt and Putnam to Parke Davis, two apparently had some side-effects. These may well be related to the direct action of the drug. The membrane-stabilizing property it has is, interestingly, as effective in the heart for controlling dysrhythmia as in the cerebral electrical disturbance associated with clinical seizures. It is possibly owing to the fact that the drug has been available for such a long time that the list of side-effects is extensive, affecting a wide variety, perhaps all, of the systems in the body.

Apart from such minor gastrointestinal problems, such as nausea and vomiting, as reported with almost any anticonvulsant, there are such features as headache, dizziness and unsteadiness. Though skin rashes of varying severity may occur, what is maybe more worrying when it is given chronically is the coarsening of the facial features that occurs, in association with acne and the growth of excess hair on the face. Another disfigurement which is very common is gum enlargement, which may become so advanced if not treated, that the teeth may almost disappear in the superabundant growth of tissue. Fortunately, this is not only treatable, but is largely preventable by careful dental hygiene. There are also effects on mental functioning in the young, with the occurrence of problems in schooling. Nevertheless, when control of seizures is paramount, phenytoin may still be the drug of choice for a particular individual.

There are, in addition, complications in the haematological system, and this may reflect the disturbance of vitamin B metabolism, particularly folic acid, leading not only to large cells in the blood, but also on occasions to disturbance of spinal and also mental functioning. Of interest here is the fact that correction of deficiencies may indeed lead to a marked worsening of seizures, implying that this control of blood levels of folic acid may, in fact, be part of the operative mechanism of the drug (see Chapter 11). Rarely, a disturbance of calcium metabolism can be severe enough to lead to weakening of the bone, and considerable pain.

WHY PHENYTOIN?

There still remains considerable mystery as to how Putnam arrived at his views concerning the phenyl radical anticonvulsant activity, even after reading his reminiscences[5]. Glazko reviewed various possibilities, including some observations that a physician colleague shared with Putnam about the muscle twitchings which occur in uraemic patients when toxic phenyls are present. It was pointed out, however, by Glazko that no clear relationship exists between phenyls and phenytoin, yet it was this apparently that was in part responsible for Putnam's leap to a phenyl containing non-hypnotic compound, related to the barbiturates. As we have noted before, once again, an incorrect hypothesis has nevertheless led to progress, perhaps because the experimenter has kept an open mind.

In conclusion, Putnam and colleagues made a major contribution to the treatment of epilepsy, and it is of interest in terms of the interplay between them and Parke Davis who, within 2 years of the discovery of the antiepileptic effect of phenytoin, had made the drug available to the medical profession for treatment under the name of Dilantin. Yet in spite of great expertise, the casino factors – luck, chance and serendipity – played their part. As Garrison[8] comments in his *History of Medicine*, 'it is no great exaggeration to say that science owes much to the shining individualism of a few chosen spirits', and he quotes the famous American neurologist, Weir Mitchell, who emphasized that 'the success of a discovery depends upon the time of its appearance'.

REFERENCES

1. Glazko, A.J. (1986). Discovery of phenytoin – historical commentary. *Therapeutic Drug Monitoring*, **8**, 490
2. Spiegel, E.A. (1937). Quantitative determination of convulsive reactivity by electrical stimulation of the brain with the skull intact. *J. Lab. Clin. Med.*, **22**, 1274
3. Merritt, H.H. and Putnam, T.J. (1945). Experimental determination of anticonvulsant activity of chemical compounds. *Epilepsia*, **3**, 51
4. Putnam, T.J. and Merritt, H.H. (1937). Experimental determination of the anticonvulsant properties of some phenyl derivatives. *Science*, **85**, 525

5.   Putnam, T.J. (1970). Demonstration of specific anticonvulsant action of diphenylhydantoin and related compounds. In Ayd, F.J. Jr. (ed.) *Discoveries in Biological Psychiatry Symposium, Baltimore.* Ayd Medical Communications, 85

6.   Merritt, H.H., Putnam T.J. and Schwab, D.M. (1937/8). A new series of anticonvulsant drugs tested by experiments on animals. *Trans. Am. Neurol.*, (1937), **62**, 123; *Am. Med. Assoc. Arch. Neurol. Psychiatry*, (1938), **39**, 1003

7.   Merritt, H.H. and Putnam, T.J. (1938). Sodium diphenylhydantoin in the treatment of convulsive disorders. *J. Am. Med. Assoc.*, **111**, 1068

8.   Garrison, F.H. (1929). *History of Medicine.* 4th edn. (Philadelphia: Saunders)

7

After phenytoin – 1937 to 1963

The discovery of phenytoin represented the third major advance in the treatment of epilepsy and it was nearly 30 years before the next drug, which still remains a first-line approach – carbamazepine – began to be used. However, there were many developments in the meantime which will be reviewed in this chapter. Some of the drugs introduced in this period such as the diones, in particular tridione, were the first effective compounds for the treatment of petit mal epilepsy. Tridione has been superseded by the succinamides, especially ethosuximide, which in its turn has been eclipsed by the appearance of sodium valproate after that of carbamazepine.

SCREENING FOR NEW EFFECTIVE DRUGS

Having developed the electric shock model in the cat, used to assess the clinically successful phenytoin[1-3], Putnam and Merritt continued to search for other substances which might be even more successful. Their animal model was shown to produce repeatable results so that test re-test data were satisfactory. A comparison was possible of the efficacy of various compounds as shown by the changes in the seizure threshold.

Out of 746 compounds tested by Merritt and Putnam[4], 76 were found to have a raised threshold without problems of toxicity. The list included not only many substances in the hydantoin series, but also diones which were part of the family of compounds which were to prove particularly useful.

The screening programmes were also adapted by other pharmaceutical companies and led to the discovery of the succinamide drugs.

97

Also about this time, there was the development of the first reliable assays of plasma concentration, so that it was possible to establish the relationship between the blood level of a drug and the therapeutic effect. This was a major step in the advance of treatment. Indeed when the assay techniques were simplified and became more generally available in the 1970s, they assisted greatly in the move towards treatment with a single compound – monotherapy. It gave the clinician confidence that the drug was actually being taken by the patient, and reached what by then were the accepted therapeutic levels for control of seizures. In parallel with these advances were the animal toxicity studies, essential as one step in the direction of providing the patient with a safe, as well as effective drug.

Other hydantoins

As a result of screening of the hydantoin series of compounds, others were introduced for treatment. Ethotoin and mephenytoin are two examples; in fact they proved to be less potent and were relatively little used. Indeed by the early 1990s, they no longer appeared in pharmaceutical listings. The same is true of phenacetamide which was discarded mainly on account of its haematological toxic effects and relatively limited potency.

TREATMENT OF PETIT MAL

The late 1940s saw the introduction of drugs that were effective in petit mal or 'absence' seizures. The first drugs were in the dione series. Although no longer used, the compound studied in detail which appeared to have been the most efficacious was trimethadione (trioxidone). This compound had been synthesized earlier by Spielman[5], in his search for a sedative and analgesic drug. It was ineffective in this respect but was of value for the petit mal type of epilepsy. The findings were confirmed by others[6], and of particular interest was the fact that it abolished the three cycles per second spike and wave in the EEG (shown to be characteristic as long ago as 1935 by Gibbs and his colleagues) (see Chapter 5, Figure 5).

Observations on trimethadione were an important advance, being a clear indication that drugs could have a selective action in various types of epilepsy, and emphasized further the concept of structure–activity relationships, which was put forward by Putnam in relation to phenytoin and has formed the basis of much subsequent pharmacological work. Further, trimethadione had relatively little effect when tested using the cat electric shock method. It did, however, control minor seizures in another animal model which was devised at this stage. Here seizures were induced by injection of various chemical agents, including most importantly the frequently used pentylene tetrazol, often called metrazol. The discovery of this model was instrumental in further research for drugs valuable in the therapy of absence seizures. In particular, the use of the succinamide group of compounds resulted.

The succinamides evolved from a systematic search for other agents that were less toxic than the diones, in particular, the oxazolidinediones. The most important compound of the series was ethosuximide. It was similar to trimethadione, being active in the chemical model with metrazol, rather than the electroshock paradigm. Studies on therapeutic effectiveness in man indicate its efficacy, often not just controlling but even abolishing petit mal seizures totally. There is rarely in medicine gain without cost and here the cost was the occurrence, perhaps the precipitation, of tonic/clonic seizures. These required treatment with other agents such as phenobarbitone or phenytoin in addition to ethosuximide. It was only with the later introduction of sodium valproate, which has a double action in controlling major and minor attacks, that monotherapy was possible.

SEIZURES IN CHILDHOOD

There are several conditions which are important causes of seizures in childhood and must be mentioned, if only briefly, in this book for completeness. The two main disorders are infantile spasms and febrile seizures. However, there are many others, neonatal seizures, including pyridoxine-dependent attacks, the Lennox Gastaut syndrome and benign childhood epilepsy in the older groups, to mention a few.

The neonatal period

Epilepsy in the young shows, not surprisingly, different patterns from that in adults. First of all neonatal seizures may be difficult to recognize clinically because they often appear in subtle forms with only apparently trivial clinical manifestations. As a result, cerebral EEG and video monitoring can be helpful[7]. Causation ranges from congenital disorders through birth injury to metabolic disorders.

One particular condition, pyridoxine-dependent seizures, is of considerable interest, because this relates directly to the neuroinhibitory transmitter, gamma-aminobutyric acid (GABA)[8]. Pyridoxine, vitamin B6, is essential as part of a co-enzyme system in the formation of GABA. Dietary deficiency may result from using certain types of processed milk and the brain GABA is depleted, only returning to normal after the diet is supplemented. The condition is genetically determined and may curiously cause convulsive movements *in utero*, of which the mother becomes aware.

If generalized convulsions occur in the first 24 hours of life, large doses of pyridoxine, 100 mg a day, 10 or 20 times the normal daily requirement, are needed to control the seizures, and the vitamin must be continued. This substance, however, probably has no place in the epilepsy of older children, but may be helpful in other rare inherited metabolic disorders.

Infantile spasms

The disorder in which salaam attacks occur very frequently, also called West's syndrome, is a very serious condition, which affects the young infant in the first months and years of life, at a stage when the brain is still maturing, hence its great impact. The condition carries a considerable mortality, and in those that survive morbidity is marked, both with continuing seizure disorder, and even more importantly in relation to retarded mental development. The EEG shows a gross abnormality (Figure 1). Detailed long-term follow-up showed that only about 10% of survivors were attending normal school and even these were functioning well below the level of their peers[9].

Conventional anticonvulsants tended to be of little value but it was the striking discovery of Sorel[10] that was responsible for the

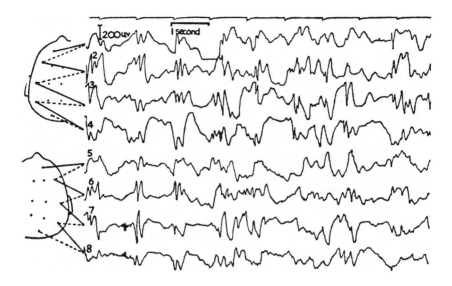

Figure 1 The EEG of hypsarrhythmia associated with infantile spasms. It shows a totally disorganized pattern, which is continuous with very high spikes, sharp waves and spikes bilaterally. This pattern is normalized by use of ACTH (see text). (Reproduced from the author's *Understanding EEG*, Duckworth, 1976)

breakthrough in treatment. It was found that adrenocorticotrophic treatment (ACTH) controlled the seizures in most cases, quite dramatically, with normalization of the EEGs. When ACTH was given early it had a beneficial effect in reducing mortality and morbidity, particularly on the psychological side.

More recently it has been shown that sodium valproate and the benzodiazepine clonazepam can also be of value in some patients, though the recurrence of this condition almost always has a serious impact.

Other types of childhood epilepsy

There are other types of epilepsy occurring in childhood[11], many of which show myoclonic jerks as a striking feature. It is an area where classification is difficult[12] and the syndromes vary from the benign to the very severe.

The names of two famous epileptologists are attached to one particular condition, the Lennox–Gastaut syndrome[13], which begins between the ages of 1 and 8 years, and is characterized by a variety of different types of seizures in which myoclonic jerks figure prominently. Status epilepticus also occurs. The EEG is markedly abnormal, attacks are difficult to control and mental retardation is often a feature.

This condition contrasts with the benign childhood epilepsy, which affects a somewhat older group. Here the fits may be very infrequent, though the EEG may show a striking picture with many complexes, often clearly focal, but without underlying structural abnormality on neuro-imaging. The seizures are usually well controlled by drugs, and disappear by the early teens, though there is a separate group, also benign, in which attacks start at that age. The prognosis is usually good, both for disappearance of seizures and mental development.

Febrile seizures

There is a long history concerning febrile convulsions. They were clearly described in the Hippocratic corpus but also earlier in Babylonian text and possibly even earlier in the ancient medical writings of India (see Chapter 2). In the seventeenth century Willis was well aware of the condition:

> 'for as much as children who fall into fevers about the time of breeding of teeth, are not all tormented with convulsions, it therefore follows that some disposition to the disease, either innate or acquired, doth proceed ...' (cited by Lennox[14])

Though fever may precipitate occasional seizures in older children and adults who have epilepsy, the term febrile seizures is reserved for attacks which occur with fever in children up to say 3 to 5 years of age. They are a common event[15]; the actual figure is controversial, but it is suggested that 5% of children have at least one convulsion in the first 5 years of life, and more than half of them are related to fever[16]. There is also a genetic disposition as Willis[17] had surmised. This inheritance is quite distinct from seizures occurring in normothermic individuals. Control of seizures, particularly if multiple, is non-controversial, for nowadays intravenous diazepam, or this drug administered rectally, is the treatment of choice.

The main point to be emphasized is that damage to the temporal lobe and the deeper structures, such as the hippocampus in particular, may occur from prolonged febrile convulsions with associated anoxia and this can lead to seizures in teenagers and adults. These attacks, which are of various types, and labelled according to the international convention as simple or partial complex seizures, may be resistant to drug treatment and require surgery (see below and Chapter 12). Hence control of febrile seizures has a major preventative role.

Studies have shown that phenobarbitone is effective in preventing repeated febrile convulsions, but its long-term use in children may lead to behaviour problems. Phenytoin is less effective, and has unwanted effects such as learning problems, as well as other manifestations of toxicity such as swollen gums which many youngsters and their families find unacceptable from a cosmetic point of view. The detailed discussion of prophylaxis is outside the scope of the present text and readers are directed to Knudsen[18]. However, it appears that treatment for febrile illness with analgesics, and in the higher risk groups sometimes combined with rectal administration of diazepam, is recommended, before the use of prolonged regular administration of anticonvulsants is contemplated.

ANTICONVULSANT PROPHYLAXIS IN ADULTS

A further matter of controversy is the prophylactic use of anticonvulsants in patients following head injury or those who have had neurosurgical treatment requiring craniotomy. There are two aspects to be considered here. The first is relatively non-controversial. It is quite clear that if seizures are a complication in the early stages following head injury, then medication with anticonvulsants is required, though for how long, and which drug should be used, are other matters presenting some difficulty. However, concerning the second point, there is some evidence that antiepileptic drugs have an effect which is quite separate from controlling seizures, namely the prevention of the development of an epileptic focus. This appears to require early introduction of the drugs, whether or not seizures have occurred, and continuation for, say, 2 years. Once again the duration of treatment, and the drugs to be chosen, and whether they should reach the accepted therapeutic level for the control of seizures, is a matter for discussion[19]. The final position in the early 1990s is yet to be established (see Chapter 11).

SOME DRUGS INTRODUCED IN THE 1950s

The barbituric acid molecule is capable of many transformations. Methylphenobarbitone (methobarbital) is one such, which had been introduced earlier and is less sedative than phenobarbitone itself. It is not widely used nowadays except, curiously, in Australia.

Primidone (Mysoline) was first synthesized by Bouge and Carrington in 1949 and was found to be effective clinically as an antiepileptic drug by Handley and Stewart[20]. It was licensed for use in 1954 in the United States and is still used in the 1990s, though not very widely. It is metabolized to phenobarbitone but in addition there are other metabolites, which have an antiepileptic action in their own right, and so may be useful in patients who are heavily sedated by phenobarbitone itself. However, primidone commonly produces troublesome side-effects especially when first used. These include dizziness and nausea, so introduction in very small doses is essential here. I personally have found that this introductory phase can be a particular problem and many patients reject the drug on the basis of their initial experience. Perhaps they share the view of none other than Napoleon Bonaparte who wrote from his island of incarceration, St Helena, in 1820: 'I do not want two diseases – one nature-made and one doctor-made'.

There are two other compounds introduced about the same time. The first is sulthiame[21] whose action is almost certainly that of blocking the metabolism of phenytoin, so levels of that drug may rise steeply when the sulthiame is introduced. The compound is now rarely used. The other, acetazolamide, which inhibits carbonic anhydrase, has already been discussed (Chapter 5) and there has recently been a resurgence of interest in adjunctive usage[22].

EPILEPSY SURGERY

There is a considerable history of the treatment of epilepsy by surgical methods. Interest in this field has fluctuated considerably; naturally activity has been concentrated at times when drug therapy was in the doldrums because of no new compounds being introduced. Such a period was that between the establishment of phenytoin as a valuable compound in the early 1940s and the introduction of carbamazepine in the late 1960s. At the present time, particularly in the light of the newer technologies, there is once again a major revival in interest.

THE EARLY HISTORY

We must begin at the beginning, though it is difficult to date just exactly when the predecessors of current day neurosurgeons started their work. Often the round regular holes in skulls of homo sapiens, that have been dated to thousands of years BC, are taken to represent the earliest examples of a surgical approach to epilepsy. It has been perhaps rather fancifully suggested that the ancients performed this trephining procedure to allow evil spirits to escape, in order to cure the seizures. Indeed this type of skull defect has been noted in much more recent specimens and suggests that the so-called primitive tribes still adhere to such a belief.

A major advance in the understanding of epilepsy in general and the role of surgery occurred in the 16th century. Ambroise Paré (1517–90) was a surgeon who became famous. He, though largely self-taught, added greatly to knowledge of the treatment of both civilian and war injuries, as well as many other conditions (Figures 2 and 3). He devised an instrument for holding the teeth apart in a convulsion (Figure 4) and treated head injuries by trephination. The following is an account of one such case, complicated by epilepsy, which was relieved:

> 'All the besieged Lords prayed me carefully to solicit above all others Monsieur de Pienne who was hurt at the breach by a stone raised by a Cannon shot in the Temple with a fracture, and depression of the bone. He told me that presently when he received the stroke, he fell to the earth as dead, and cast blood out of his mouth, nose and ears with great vomitings, and was fourteen days without speaking one word, or having any reason; there happened to him also startings somewhat like Convulsions, and had all his face swell'd and livid. He was trepan'd on the side of the temporal muscle upon the Os Coronale. I dressed him with other Chirurgions, and God cured him, and is at this day living, God be thanked'[23].

A very characteristic ending to many of Paré's case histories.

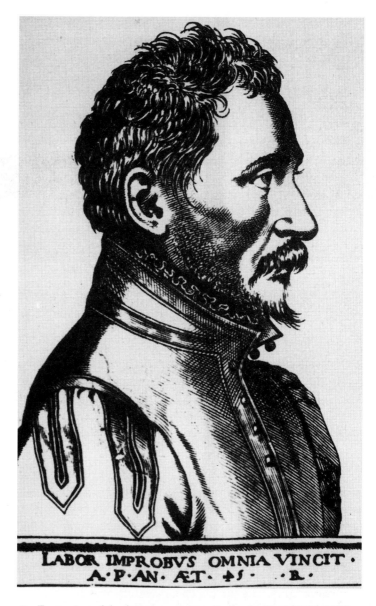

Figure 2 Engraving of the famous surgeon, Ambroise Paré (1517–1590), aged 45 years, in the Hunterian Collection of the University of Glasgow. His works include the '*Apologie and Treatise*', containing 'Voyages Made into Diverse Places', 'Account of the Plague', 'Discussions on Gunshot Wounds' and the 'Surgical Aphasias and Rules'. Title page of Paré's *Anatomie Universelle*, Paris, 1561

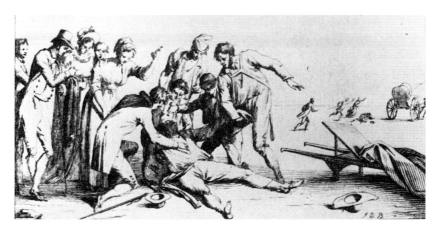

Figure 3 'The Epileptic' by Jean Duplessi-Bertaux (1774–1819). (Reproduced with kind permission from The Henry Barton Jacobs Collection of John Hopkins University)

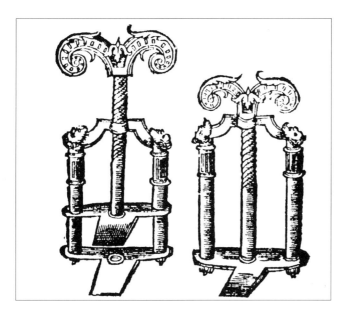

Figure 4 Instrument of the 16th century surgeon Ambroise Paré, called the 'Speculum Oris', used to overcome contraction of the jaws that occurred during seizures, in order to prevent tongue biting. This device would almost certainly damage the teeth, and nowadays even the padded spoon of more recent times has been replaced (from Paré's collected works, 4th edn., 1585)

THE MODERN BEGINNINGS

The true beginning of surgery of epilepsy, however, dates to the latter half of the nineteenth century. William MacEwen, Rickman Godlee and Victor Horsley all played an important part in the advances. It was Godlee who performed the first recorded operation for a cerebral glioma[24] whilst the honour of the first direct treatment of epilepsy must go to Victor Horsley (1857–1918). Surgery had advanced by the use of general anaesthesia, mainly chloroform, and aseptic surgical conditions, as well as a fuller understanding of cerebral localization. By the time Horsley was appointed Surgeon to the staff of the Hospital for Paralysed and Epileptics, Queen's Square, in 1886, he had probably performed more than 100 experimental cranial operations in monkeys[24]. In this work he established surgical protocols for wound asepsis, general anaesthesia and the types of skull flaps and methods of bone removal. The use of irrigation with hot solutions and the application of bone wax was also examined in these studies.

During his first year at Queen's Square he performed ten intracranial operations including one on a patient of Hughlings Jackson where a cortical scar was removed in an attempt to control epilepsy.

Case history

The patient was a man of 22 years of age who had developed epilepsy 7 years previously. The seizures were intractable and resulted from a compound fracture of the skull at the age of 7 years. Remarkably he had 3000 fits in 14 days prior to the operation and this was associated with not only overall mental deterioration, but also a Todd's paralysis, weakness affecting the left arm and leg. The details of the operation with diagrams are still available in the hospital records (cited by Thomas[24]). After the procedure the patient was greatly improved, not only in relation to seizures and the hemiparesis, but also his psychological state.

Horsley continued to expand his surgical interest, performing, for example, laminectomies. He also became involved in political matters, even standing for Parliament in 1910. Horsley was unsuccessful and this is probably because he supported the idea of votes for women. Further, he did not dissociate himself from the militant aspects of the suffragette campaign, and as a result he was not elected.

THE LATER HISTORY OF NEUROSURGERY IN EPILEPSY

Advances in the neurosurgery of epilepsy depended not only on the EEG for the localization of seizure discharge, but also on neuroimaging techniques for the detection of lesions, whether, for example, scars or tumours. The introduction of antibiotics for the control of sepsis was another important matter. Pioneering work was carried out by Wilder Penfield and colleagues at the Montreal Neurological Institute[25] and by Murray Falconer and associates[26] at the Guys–Maudsley Neurosurgical Unit in London, a little later. As a result partly of experience, the techniques became safe and more effective in their seizure control. Approximately two-thirds of patients were either fit-free or had a very marked reduction in seizure frequency.

Though neurosurgical techniques have continued to be used for many years, interest switched to more effective anticonvulsants, but the 1980s have seen a resurgence of neurosurgery. This has been linked with the introduction of EEG ambulatory monitoring with various telemetric techniques combined with video monitoring. The placement of intracranial electrodes and subsequent prolonged records for hours or days have allowed much more accurate localization of the site of origin of seizure discharges. Currently in the early 1990s (see Chapter 12) these more complex methods of evaluation and the advancement in surgical techniques have been paralleled by the introduction of newer anticonvulsant compounds such as vigabatrin and lamotrigine. The former has a direct effect on the synthesis, course of action and breakdown of gamma-aminobutyric acid (GABA), the most important CNS inhibitory substance. This part of the story is continued in Chapters 11 and 12.

REFERENCES

1. Putnam, T.J. and Merritt, H.H. (1937). Experimental determination of the anticonvulsant properties of some phenyl derivatives. *Science*, **85**, 525
2. Merritt, H.H. and Putnam, T.J. (1938). Sodium diphenylhydantoin in the treatment of convulsive disorders. *J. Am. Med. Assoc.*, **111**, 1068
3. Merritt, H.H. and Putnam, T.J. (1940). Further experiences with the use

of sodium diphenylhydantoin in the treatment of convulsive disorders. *Am. J. Psychiatry*, **96**, 1023

4. Merritt, H.H. and Putnam, T.J. (1945). Experimental determination of anticonvulsant activity of chemical compounds. *Epilepsia*, **3**, 51

5. Spielman, M.A. (1944). Some analgesic agents derived from oxozolidine 2-4-dione. *J. Am. Chem. Soc.*, **66**, 1244

6. Goodman, L., Toman, J. and Swinyard, E. (1946). The anticonvulsant properties of Tridione: laboratory and clinical investigations. *Am. J. Med.*, **1**, 213

7. Tuchman, R.F. and Moshe, S.L. (1990). Neonatal seizures: diagnostic and treatment controversies. In Sillanpää, M., Johannessen, S.I., Blennow, G. and Dam, M. (eds.) *Psychiatric Epilepsy*. (Petersfield, UK: Wrightson)

8. Brown, J.K. (1982). Fits in children. In Laidlaw, J. and Richens, A. (eds.) *Textbook of Epilepsy*. (Edinburgh: Churchill Livingstone)

9. Jeavons, P.M., Bower, D.P. and Dimitrakondi, M. (1973). Long-term prognosis of 150 cases of 'West's Syndrome'. *Epilepsia*, **14**, 153

10. Sorel, L. and Dusaucy-Bauloye, A. (1958). A propos de 21 cas d'hypsarythmie de Gibbs. Son traitement spectaculaire par l'ACTH. *Acta Neurolog. Belg.*, **58**, 130

11. Aicardi, J. (1988). Epileptic syndromes in childhood. *Epilepsia*, **29**, 51

12. Commission of Classification and Terminology of the ILAE. (1989). Proposal for revised classification of epilepsies and epileptic syndromes, **30**, 389

13. Beaumanoir, A. (1985). The Lennox-Gastaut Syndrome. In Roper, J., Dravet, C., Bureau, M., Dreifuss, F.E. and Wolf, P. (eds.) *Epileptic Syndromes*. (London and Paris: Libbey)

14. Lennox, W.G. (1960). *Epilepsy and Convulsive Disorders*. (Boston: Little Brown)

15. Annegers, J.F., Hauser, W.A., Shirts, S.B. and Kurland, L.T. (1987). Factors prognostic of unprovoked seizures after febrile convulsions. *New Engl. J. Med.*, **316**, 493

16. Wallace, S.J. (ed.) (1988). *The Child with Febrile Seizures*. (London: Butterworths)

17. Willis, I. (1685). The London practice of physick. In *The Whole Practical Part of Physick*. (London: George and Crooke)

18. Knudsen, F.U. (1990). Febrile convulsions. In Sillanpää, M., Johannessen, S., Blenow, G. and Dam, M. (eds.) *Paediatric Epilepsy*. (Petersfield, UK: Wrightson)

19. Jennett, B. (1982). Post-traumatic epilepsy. In Laidlaw, J. and Richens, A. (eds.) *A Textbook of Epilepsy*. (Edinburgh: Churchill Livingstone)

20. Handley, R. and Stewart, A.S.R. (1952). Mysoline: a new drug in the treatment of epilepsy. *Lancet*, **262**, 742

21. Green, J.R., Troupin, A.S., Halpern, L.M., Friel, P. and Kanarek, P. (1974). Suthiame: evaluation as an anti-convulsant. *Epilepsia*, **15**, 329
22. Oles, K.S., Penry, J.K., Cole, D.L.W. and Howard, G. (1989). Use of acetazolamide as an adjunct to carbamazepine in refractory partial seizures. *Epilepsia*, **30**, 74
23. Paré, Ambroise. (1575). *Apologie and Treatise containing The Voyages Made into Diverse Places, with many writings upon surgery*
24. Thomas, G.D.T. (1989). The first generation of neurosurgeons. In Rose, F.C. (ed.) *Neuroscience Across the Centuries*. (London: Smith-Gordon)
25. Penfield, W. and Jasper, H. (1954). *Epilepsy and the Functional Anatomy of the Human Brain*. (Boston: Little Brown)
26. Falconer, M.A. (1965). The surgical treatment of temporal lobe epilepsy. *Neurochirurgia*, **8**, 160

8

Carbamazepine

Almost 100 years had elapsed from the introduction of bromides to the time when carbamazepine emerged, and about 50 years after the introduction of phenobarbitone. In the interim, drugs strongly active in petit mal epilepsy, the succinamides, were added to the pharmacy shelves. Different companies and countries had contributed so far to the drug treatment of epilepsy, the countries being Britain, the USA and Germany.

It was another company and another country that was responsible for the discovery of carbamazepine, namely Geigy in Switzerland.

THE SEARCH FOR A NEW PSYCHOTROPIC DRUG

The story begins with an attempt to find analogues for chlorpromazine. This was first introduced in 1952, and proved to be one of the most active psychotropic drugs for schizophrenia and states in which over-activity occurs, for example, mania. In spite of the fact that newer compounds emerged, both for oral and depot administration, it still remains an important therapeutic agent.

During the early 1950s a search for an even more effective psychotropic drug was under way in many pharmaceutical firms all over the world. Cynics may regard this type of pursuit as merely an effort to produce a 'me too' compound, in order to siphon off profits from the companies which had completed the basic research. Nevertheless, in the case of the work of Geigy in Basle, it was to prove extremely valuable, as has been the case in other such detailed searches with meticulous screening by many companies and individual chemists.

113

CARBAMAZEPINE DISCOVERED

In 1953 chemists synthesized the first in the series of carbamoyl compounds that subsequently yielded carbamazepine[1]. It had a urea ring in the structure, and interestingly bore more similarities to the antidepressants such as imipramine, than to the phenothiazines. This psychotropic aspect has proved to be of considerable interest, in addition to the antiepileptic properties. These were soon recognized and first demonstrated in experimental animals, and were to produce the most profound change in the treatment of patients with seizure disorders. Carbamazepine had effects against electro-induced seizures in mice and rats, and metrazol-induced seizures in mice. A variety of other animal models also demonstrated the effectiveness of this drug, either with chemically or electrically induced fits.

These pharmacological effects in animals resemble phenytoin in many ways. However, carbamazepine is more effective than phenytoin in reducing stimulus-induced discharges in rats, as well as blocking chemically induced seizures[2], and reduces the kindling effect (see Chapter 11). Like the hydantoins the carbamoyl compounds act in the rat amygdala[3,4] and on many systems in the body. Apart from controlling the pain of trigeminal neuralgia, some have a local anaesthetic action; whilst carbamazepine itself is antidiuretic and can be used in the treatment of diabetes insipidus. It also has a place in cardiology because of its antiarrhythmic effects.

CLINICAL USE

Theobald and Kunz[5] were able to report a characteristic pattern of activity, and the first clinical trials were quickly undertaken demonstrating its efficacy. The drug was introduced under the trade name, Tegretol®, in Switzerland the same year. The observation that carbamazepine was effective in trigeminal neuralgia was made concurrently[6].

Early on in the clinical studies it was observed that improvement in the patient's mental state might occur; depressive symptoms, particularly if they had been exaggerated by the use of phenobarbitone, would lift and there was general improvement in well-being. Indeed, the use specifically for psychotropic actions (see below) has more recently been recognized[7].

114

Carbamazepine is generally well tolerated with relatively minor side-effects reported[8], especially if begun at low dosage. It could, however, be regarded as having a 'slow start' in some countries, including the US, because of potentially more serious toxicity. Among the reasons were the early reports of serious blood dyscrasias. One of the problems is the action of carbamazepine, soon after it is first prescribed, in reducing leukocyte counts in some patients. The level of the reduction is sufficient to be a concern to haematologists, who suggest that the drug should be stopped at once. This change in the blood count, which may in part have accounted for some of the initial resistance to the use of carbamazepine, is no real cause for concern, because the effect is transitory. Since the early days there now seem fewer reports of serious haematological complications, and it is available worldwide. Carbamazepine can also interfere with water and electrolyte homeostasis[9]. It causes hyponatraemia in 10–15% of patients, but is seldom symptomatic or severe enough to produce fluid retention.

PSYCHOTROPIC ACTION

Soon after carbamazepine was introduced, the beneficial effects on the mental state of patients were reported. In a review of published papers[10], it was noted that the majority of authors indicated such an effect. Not only was there a clear-cut improvement in behaviour, with increased speed of bodily movements and in psychic processing, but also obvious elevation of mood. These findings, at first relatively anecdotal, were confirmed by controlled investigations in which comparisons were made with other drugs, employing detailed measurements by rating scales (see Trimble[11] for review).

PSYCHIATRIC DISORDER IN EPILEPSY

The observations on the value of carbamazepine highlighted the importance of associated psychiatric disorders in patients with epilepsy. This is a topic with a long history, and full discussion is outside the scope of this book. However, some points in this controversial area require mention. It is first of all most important to emphasize that epilepsy is not linked to any specific psychiatric or behavioural syndrome, and though it may be associated with, for example, mental retardation, the seizures are part of the congenital or acquired condition responsible for both.

Depressive illness

The most common disturbance currently found in patients with epilepsy between seizures, is of a depressive nature[12]. In the earlier literature, in fact until quite recently, the term melancholia has been used, and the condition was observed even in antiquity, including by Hippocrates. Later Aretaeus noted that not only was there languor and unsociability present, but also disturbance of sleep and appetite[13]. All these are recognized as indicating a true depressive illness, while Griesinger[14] emphasized that melancholia could be associated with suicidal tendencies.

Clearly the patient with epilepsy has a considerable burden, because it not only affects, for example, work and leisure, but usually requires constant and long-continued medication which may produce troublesome side-effects. It has recently been shown that these are greatly reduced if only one antiepileptic drug is given, that is, mono-therapy is adopted[15]. In theory, treatment of depression presents a problem because virtually all antidepressants are convulsant in addition. Fortunately in the clinical situation, if they are introduced at low dosage with smaller incremental elevations, seizures are rarely augmented and the depressive condition can be alleviated.

Schizophrenia and epilepsy

The relationship of schizophreniform psychosis to epilepsy has been recognized for many years. For example, Falret writing in the mid-nineteenth century had given a clear description of the disorder[16]. The neurologist, Hughlings Jackson[17] said that epilepsy was 'a cause of insanity in 6% of insane persons'. Later a notable German psychiatrist, Kraepelin, in 1922 in a definitive textbook on psychiatry[18], regarded the main groupings of psychiatric illness as manic depressive insanity, dementia praecox (what is now called schizophrenia), and epileptic insanity.

More recently, the relationship between schizophrenia and epilepsy was studied extensively by Slater and Beard[19], and by Trimble[20]. The features of the schizophrenic illness associated with epilepsy are not dissimilar to other types, except that the age of onset tends to be later, personality is preserved and rapport with others, including doctors, is maintained. Oddly, the onset of the psychosis occurs when the attacks, usually of temporal lobe type, are well controlled.

It is intriguing, however, that there appears to be an antagonism between epilepsy and schizophrenia, and this is often given as the reason why convulsive therapy was introduced into psychiatric practice for the treatment of psychosis. In particular, it is often suggested that von Meduna was responsible for this, because he observed such an antagonism between the two conditions, epilepsy and schizophrenia. The matter is controversial, but it seems more likely that it was not the dissociation of the two conditions themselves, but the fact that psychiatric symptoms in some patients were improved if seizures occurred.

There is another intriguing inverse relationship that has been noted, namely the fact that the EEG may be normal at the time of onset of psychosis, the so-called 'forced normalization', while it is known to show disturbance at other times. This pattern first noted by Landolt[21], though it does occur, is in my experience less frequent than the pattern one might expect on general grounds, namely the worsening of the EEG abnormality, in some patients with seizures, at the onset of psychosis.

Left versus right hemisphere disturbance

Psychological differences are present between the hemispheres in terms of function. Apart from verbal and related tasks being the responsibility of the left hemisphere in the majority of individuals, it has been relatively difficult to establish what exactly are right hemisphere functions. A distinguished neurologist, chairing a symposium on this subject at a conference, observed that the left hemisphere could be likened to the city of Berlin, an active, bustling crossing point, whilst the right hemisphere in contrast – Vienna – had a relationship to culture, and particularly music. It is well known that ability in the latter respect is a feature of right hemisphere function. Another difference concerns certain pathological conditions; damage to the left hemisphere appears more likely to lead to epilepsy when this is predominantly on the left rather than the right side[22].

117

One who explored the relationship of psychosis to epilepsy was Flor-Henry[23], who introduced a new and intriguing vista. He showed that a left-sided temporal EEG abnormality, particularly, was likely to be associated with a schizophreniform psychosis, and he regarded the right as being important in relation to manic depressive psychosis. In fact Robertson[24] considered a right-sided focus as a predisposing factor in those patients with depressive illness. However, in general this finding has not been confirmed, whilst there is considerable evidence from various spheres of the main observation of Flor-Henry, about the particular importance of left-sided disturbance in relation to schizophrenia. Evidence from electroencephalography, radiology, psychometry and symptom check lists has all pointed strongly in this direction. Of further interest has been the observation that, for example, male schoolchildren with a left-sided focus, and treated with phenytoin, may show both greater behavioural problems and poorer scholastic performance than with right hemisphere lesions[25]. There is also a growing body of evidence which points to the importance of laterality of abnormality in non-epileptic psychiatric patients[26].

PSYCHOTROPIC ACTIONS OF CARBAMAZEPINES

As mentioned earlier, carbamazepine has a multitude of actions, and though the observation of improvement for behaviour and mood in patients with epilepsy was noted very early on in its use, employing the drugs specifically in a psychiatric context for patients without epilepsy, is more recent. Its applications are largely in manic depressive psychosis[27]. Interestingly, it is particularly effective in the manic phase of such disorders, where controlled studies have shown that the value is not dissimilar to that of lithium. It may also be used in the treatment of depressive illness, though its place in this respect is not established.

In psychiatric practice, perhaps the most important drug that could be discovered is one which prevents the onset of manic or depressive episodes in those who have bipolar depression, or prevents the depressive episodes in those who have the unipolar state. Lithium is well established in this respect, but side-effects are considerable and stabilization of the patient on the drug may prove difficult. Carbamazepine does have positive effects in this context, and its actions, though perhaps not as marked as those of lithium, are significant because of the ease of instituting treatment and the relative lack of side-effects.

CONCLUSION

Carbamazepine is notable in that soon after being synthesized, it was found to be antiepileptic, and only a short time elapsed before its clinical use. It is of interest that the drug regulatory authorities may increase the interval between these phases. This has been exemplified particularly by the case of carbamazepine, where the US Food and Drug Administration (the FDA) did not approve of the use in epilepsy until 1974, almost 10 years after its introduction in Europe, whereas the FDA had earlier permitted its use in the treatment of trigeminal neuralgia. Yet in the 1990s it is still certainly a first-line drug, now also available in a slow-release form; it is available worldwide for 150 countries under several confusingly different trade names.

REFERENCES

1. Schindler, W. and Häfliger, F. (1954). Uber Derivate des Iminodibenzyls. *Helv. Chim. Acta*, **37**, 472
2. Rall, T.W. and Schleifer, L.S. (1985). Drugs effective in the treatment of epilepsy. In Goodman, L.S. and Gilman, A.G. *Pharmacological Basis of Therapeutics*, 7th edn. (London: MacMillan)
3. Albright, P.S. (1983). Effects of carbamazepine, clonazepam and phenytoin on seizure threshold in amygdala and cortex. *Exp. Neurol.*, **79**, 11
4. Albright, P.S. and Burnham, W.M. (1980). Development of a new pharmacological seizure model: effects of anticonvulsants on cortical and amygdala-kindled seizure in rats. *Epilepsia*, **21**, 681
5. Theobald, W. and Kunz, H.A. (1963). Zur Phamakologie des Antiepilepticums 5, Carbomyl-5H-dibenzo(bf)azepin. *Arzneimittelforschung*, **13**, 122
6. Bloom, S. (1962). Trigeminal neuralgia: its treatment with a new anticonvulsant drug (G32883). *Lancet*, **1**, 839
7. Post, R.M., Uhde, T.W., Rubinow, D.R., Ballenger, J.C. and Gold, P.W. (1983). Biochemical effects of carbamazepine; relationship to its mechanisms of action in affective illness. *Prog. Neuropsychol. Pharmacol. Biol. Psychiatry*, **7**, 263
8. Livingstone, S., Pauli, L.L. and Berman, W. (1974). Carbamazepine in epilepsy. *Dis. Nerv. Syst.*, **35**, 103

9. Mucklow, J. (1991). Selected side-effects: 2. Carbamazepine and hyponatraemia. *Prescribers J.*, **31**, 61
10. Dalby, M.A. (1975). Behavioural effects of carbamazepine. In Penry, J.K. and Daly, D.D. (eds.) *Advances in Neurology*. (New York: Raven Press)
11. Trimble, M.R. (1987). Antiepileptic and psychotropic properties of carbamazepine. In Crawford, R. and Silverstone, T. (eds.) *Carbamazepine in Affective Disorders*. (London: Clinical Neuroscience Publishers)
12. Betts, T.A., Mersky, H. and Pond, D.A. (1976). Psychiatry. In Laidlaw, J. and Richens, A. (eds.) *A Textbook of Epilepsy*. (London: Churchill Livingstone)
13. Temkin, O. (1945). *The Falling Sickness*. (Baltimore: Johns Hopkins Press) (2nd edn., 1971, New York: Dover)
14. Griesinger, W. (1857). *Mental Pathology and Therapeutics*. Translated Lockhart, Robertson and Rutherford. (London: J. New Sydenham Society)
15. Reynolds, E.H., Elwes, R.D.C. and Shovon, S.D. (1983). Why does epilepsy become intractable? Prevention of chronic epilepsy. *Lancet*, **2**, 952
16. Falret, J. (1860). De l'état mental des épileptiques. *Arch. Gen. Med.*, **16**, 661
17. Hughlings Jackson, J. (1875–1880). Temporary mental disorders after epileptic paroxysms. *West Riding Lunatic Asylum Medical Report*, **5**, 1875–80
18. Kraepelin, E. (1922). *Psychiatrie*, Vol 3, 8th edn. (Leipzig: Johan Abrosium Barth)
19. Slater, E. and Beard, A.W. (1963). The schizophrenia-like psychosis of epilepsy. *Br. J. Psychiatry*, **95**, 109
20. Trimble, M.R. (1991). *The Psychoses of Epilepsy*. (London: Raven Press)
21. Landolt, H. (1958). Serial electroencephalographic investigations during psychotic episodes in epileptic patients and during schizophrenic attacks. In de Haas, L. (ed.) *Lectures on Epilepsy*. (London: Elsevier)
22. Scott, D.F. (1985). Left and right cerebral hemisphere differences in the occurrence of epilepsy. *Br. J. Med. Psychol.*, **58**, 189
23. Flor-Henry, P. (1969). Psychosis and temporal lobe epilepsy: a controlled investigation. *Epilepsia*, **10**, 363
24. Robertson, M.M. (1985). Depression in patients with epilepsy: an overview and clinical study. In Trimble, M.R. (ed.) *The Psychopharmacology of Epilepsy*. (Chichester, UK: Wiley)
25. Stores, G. (1978). School children with epilepsy at risk for learning and behavioural problems. *Dev. Med. Child. Neurol.*, **20**, 502
26. Taylor, M.A., Greenspan, B. and Abrams, R. (1979). Lateralised neuropsychiatric dysfunction in affective disorder and schizophrenia. *Am. J. Psychiatry*, **135**, 1031
27. Crawford, R. and Silverstone, T. (1987). Carbamazepine in affective disorder. *Int. Clin. Pharmacol.*, **2**, Suppl. 1

9

Status epilepticus and the benzodiazepines

STATUS EPILEPTICUS

In the ancient texts on epilepsy, the view was often expressed that epilepsy was not dangerous (for example in the Hippocratic corpus). Yet by the end of the nineteenth century, it had been noted that the condition of status epilepticus in which seizures of a major type followed one another without consciousness being regained, carried (and indeed still does carry) a significant mortality[1]. It was Hunter[2] in 1959 who emphasized that it was very rarely reported before Locock[3] had shown success with bromides. Thus, paradoxically, the introduction of effective treatments, potassium bromide and phenobarbitone, seems to have produced a new and serious condition.

Early recognition of status epilepticus

There are, nevertheless, a few earlier reports. The physician, Thomas Willis[4], who originated the term 'neurology', writing in 1667, commented that fits 'if oft repeated' tended to become more severe and lead to death. Sydenham, in 1689, was aware that status epilepticus, as we know it, could occur. He says:

> 'One fit comes on as fast as the other is gone, especially when the infant is almost worn out with that which is common to them all when there is a distance between them, that as soon as the fit is off they fall asleep, and continue very drowsy, and sometimes do wake in another fit.'[5].

The French used the term 'état de mal' for status epilepticus and were aware of the seriousness of the condition. In the first half of the nineteenth century, Prichard[6], in his treatise *Diseases of the Nervous System*, not only noted that there was a danger in the succession of fits without recovery of consciousness, but he also described a complication of status epilepticus, namely hemiplegia, which now goes under the eponym of Todd's paralysis. The distinguished physician Richard Bright[7], known for his particular interest in renal disease, in fact wrote a book on *Diseases of the Brain and Nervous System*, published in 1831. This contained accounts of patients who died as a result of epilepsy. It is perhaps surprising that the extensive studies towards the end of the nineteenth century, by Radcliffe[8] and Reynolds[9], did not report status epilepticus, although others at about the same time almost certainly were aware of such an occurrence. It is mentioned in the writings of doctors who worked with the mentally disturbed in the County Asylums which were gradually being established in the nineteenth century. Manley[10] in 1858 recorded that epilepsy occurred in the advanced stages of general paralysis of the insane, and a series of convulsions could be a terminal event, though the term 'status epilepticus' appeared in English for the first time only in 1867. This was in a translation of Trousseau's lectures on clinical medicine[11].

Causes of status epilepticus

Soon after the introduction of bromides in treatment, it became appreciated that their rapid withdrawal could lead to precipitation of this condition. No less a figure than Hughlings Jackson indicated, in 1870, that bromide should be reduced gradually, and not stopped suddenly as seizures were an almost certain result[12].

From this time onwards, status epilepticus was recorded in neurological writings, for example, Gowers[13], who however, regarded it as a rare occurrence outside the asylum. Aldren Turner published his comprehensive book on epilepsy in 1907[14], and observed that, though many patients did not ever have status epilepticus, some might have repeated closely spaced attacks, often known as serial seizures and yet for most of the time be relatively fit-free otherwise (Figure 1). He also noted that it might supervene in long-standing cases of epilepsy for no apparent reason, but occasionally, for some, was the first manifestation

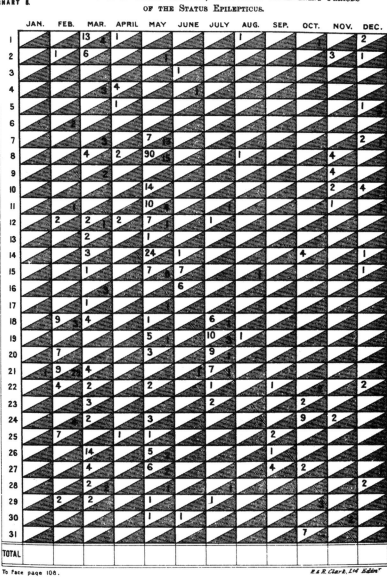

Figure 1 Fit chart from Aldren Turner's book[14], showing a severe case of epilepsy with both serial fits and status epilepticus. This actual chart is still used by some physicians, though a great variety of 'diaries', log books, etc. have been designed more recently for various purposes

123

of what was to become a chronic disorder. Clearly he was aware that the sudden cessation of bromides was a cause of status, and that it could occur after head injury; also that it could be a complication of febrile illness or toxic states.

Following the introduction of barbiturates in 1912, it soon became common knowledge that even in non-epileptic patients, when this medication was stopped abruptly, withdrawal seizures could result. For patients who already had chronic epilepsy, discontinuing the medication, either under medical instructions, or as quite often happened, of their own volition, could precipitate status epilepticus. Following the introduction of phenytoin in 1937, it was noted that status epilepticus could result from rapid withdrawal of this compound, although with subsequently prescribed compounds such as primidone, troxidone and mesantoin, this complication was less likely.

Treatment

It was in 1924 that paraldehyde was introduced as a treatment for this condition, and drastically reduced mortality. Later intramuscular phenobarbitone or intravenous phenytoin were used[15], but it became quite quickly appreciated that benzodiazepines, particularly intravenous diazepam, were extremely effective in this condition[16] and indeed still have prime position. The patient is unconscious, and may remain so even after control of seizures, so clearly intensive medical and nursing care are of crucial importance in markedly reducing the morbidity. The overall management of status epilepticus is clearly outside the scope of this book. It is reviewed by Brodie[17]. The drugs, apart from the use of the standard medications already mentioned, may include chlormethiazole and lignocaine, both of which have no particular place in the treatment of epilepsy otherwise.

In spite of these therapeutic effects, the seriousness of convulsive status epilepticus was emphasized as recently as 1970 by Rowan and Scott[1], but subsequently I have observed a decline in this disorder as well as in Todd's paralysis. The condition has tended to become the province of the neurosurgeon associated with head injury, rather than presenting to the neurologist as a cause for emergency admission. When this is the case, poor compliance is the suspect, or it may occur with too abrupt an alteration or reduction in medication, especially when phenobarbitone is involved.

BENZODIAZEPINES

Though the use of benzodiazepines in status epilepticus is of great significance, these drugs have much value in various areas in medicine. Of particular interest is their site of action. It has been shown that benzodiazepine receptors in the central nervous system are closely related to gamma-aminobutyric acid (GABA) action sites. Their pharmacological effects apart from being anticonvulsant are anxiolytic, hypnotic, muscle relaxant and amnesia producing, in order of importance (Table 1). Depending on the particular molecular configuration, they have a greater or lesser value in relation to one or other of these actions, and may have different effects depending on the route of administration. The actual dosage given is also important. Thus diazepam, a 1–4 compound, is potent as an antiepileptic drug given intravenously, but by the oral route, though it has excellent effects in terms of reducing anxiety, its impact on seizures is much less, usually transient, lasting a few days or weeks. In contrast, clobazam, a 1–5 compound, though having some anxiety reducing elements, is a potent anticonvulsant given orally. Clonazepam is another one of the series widely employed orally. It is particularly valuable in myoclonic epilepsy, but by intravenous route it can be used in status epilepticus.

Table 1 Benzodiazepine actions. The larger the number of benzodiazepine receptors occupied, the greater the degree of sedation and muscle uncoordination

Anxiolytic effect	Motor impairment
Antiepileptic action	Muscle relaxation
Hypnotic effect	Loss of consciousness
Amnesia	

The discovery of benzodiazepines

By the 1950s pharmacological chemists were well aware of the relationship between molecular structure and therapeutic action. Also, animal models for screening drugs for psychotropic effects were well established. When the uninitiated inspect chemical formulae,

125

there appear to be only a relatively small number of changes that could be performed to yield another drug in the series. This is in fact quite wrong, for with barbiturates as many as 2500 variations have been prepared, and of these, 50 have been distributed commercially. There are over 3000 compounds in the benzodiazepine series, and 120 are clinically active, and 25 of these have been marketed, taking the world as a whole. Some have a limited distribution and are only available in a small number of countries. Though some members of the series such as diazepam and nitrazepam are available internationally, they are often, confusingly, supplied under different trade names.

Chlordiazepoxide (Librium®) was the first tranquillizer to come on to the market and be widely prescribed. It was introduced by Sternbach in 1957, though it was preceded by other psychotropic drugs, which had been shown to have a taming effect on animals, notably chlorpromazine. Its antipsychotic action, particularly in schizophrenia, was known from 1952 onwards. The first use was quite different from its later established place in psychiatry. During the Indo-Chinese war, the French surgeons employed chlorpromazine in the so-called 'lytic cocktail'. It was given to battle casualties who were severely shocked, producing the effects of hypothermia and deep anaesthesia. Although no longer used for this purpose, it is still a valuable compound for the management of psychiatric patients, particularly those who are overactive. Nowadays phenothiazines are often used in depot preparations given every 2–4 weeks, often preventing relapses for many years.

Site of action

The benzodiazepine receptors are strategically placed to affect GABA binding sites, and as a result potentiate its inhibitory action (see Figure 2). There is another close spatial association in the brain receptors between benzodiazepine and barbiturate action, yet their anticonvulsive effects chemically seem dissimilar. The other consequences of benzodiazepines (Table 1), which in some circumstances are regarded as toxic manifestations, for example, excessive sedation, when anticonvulsant action is what is desired, remain to be explained.

Another rather difficult matter concerns the paradoxical action of a particular benzodiazepine, namely diazepam. On occasions, instead of

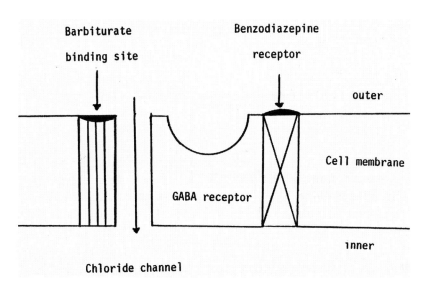

Figure 2 Schematic diagram of the arrangement of receptor sites, drawn from various sources. Note, in particular, the dose relationship of the GABA receptor to both barbiturate and benzodiazepine sites and the chloride channel. (Redrawn by the author from several sources)

controlling petit mal status, it may convert this into that of convulsive type[18,19], requiring medication of other kinds, even anaesthesia, to control the clinical manifestations which are not self-limiting.

Problems of dependency

A further problem of benzodiazepine use is the question of dependence, amounting to addiction. It is now appreciated to be a major worldwide problem, great difficulties arising in certain but not all individuals when attempts are made to curtail the dosage. Psychological symptoms appear in a gross fashion, typical physical withdrawal feelings such as tremulousness, may be profound, and these are coupled with marked recrudescence of the type of anxiety symptoms for which the drug was originally prescribed.

The situation has reached serious proportions in recent times, with legal actions pending, not only against the prescribing doctors, but also the manufacturing companies involved. It is not fully appreciated that substitution of benzodiazepines for barbiturates has been responsible for a decrease in the number of suicides by reduction in usage of the latter, which is clearly an advance. The long half-life of barbiturates, such as phenobarbitone, is particularly troublesome in the management of suicidal overdose. Now benzodiazepines have fallen into disfavour, and the search for other types of tranquillizers is proceeding apace.

The various problems arising from the use and misuse of medication were foreseen much earlier on. The comment of the sixteenth century physician, Paracelsus (1493–1541), seems appropriate here. He regards no substance as being devoid of poisonous effects, but the actual dose administered was the key to the particular substance being toxic. Certainly increased doses of tranquillizers, beyond the usual levels, cause great problems when reduction and eventual discontinuation are attempted. As a result the search for non-benzodiazepine tranquillizers has partially been successful. Already some compounds are available, though their efficacy is not entirely proven, and they are costly, as always with new compounds. Absolute statements about their likelihood to lead to dependence are not possible because of the short periods of safety testing.

In conclusion, benzodiazepines are an interesting group of substances in relation to their central nervous system site of action and their antiepileptic properties, and they particularly remain the treatment of choice by parenteral means, in status epilepticus. There are also certain members of the series, such as clonazepam and clobazam, that have value as oral preparations.

REFERENCES

1. Rowan, A.J. and Scott, D.F. (1970). Major status epilepticus. *Acta Neurol. Scand.*, **46**, 573
2. Hunter, R.A. (1959/60). Status epilepticus, history, incidence and problems. *Epilepsia*, **1**, 162
3. Locock, C. (1857). Discussion of paper by E.H. Sieveking. Analysis of fifty two cases of epilepsy observed by the author. *Lancet*, **1**, 527
4. Willis, T. (1685). The London practice of physick. In *The Whole Practical Part of Physick*. (London: George and Crook)
5. Sydenham, T. (1689). Cited by Hunter, see reference 2
6. Prichard, J.C. (1822). *A Treatise on Diseases of the Nervous System*. (London: Underwood)

7. Bright, R. (1831). *Diseases of the Brain and Nervous System*.
8. Radcliffe, C.B. (1861). *Epileptic and Other Convulsive Affections of the Nervous System, their Pathology and Treatment*. 3rd edn. (London: Churchill) (1st edn. 1854)
9. Reynolds, Sir J.R. (1861). *Epilepsy; its Symptoms, Treatment and Relation to Other Chronic Convulsive Disorders*. (London: Churchill)
10. Manley, J. (1858). On epilepsy. *J. Mental Sci.*, **4**, 245
11. Trousseau, A. (1867). Lectures on clinical medicine. Translated Bagire. *J. New Sydenham Society, London*, **1**, 53
12. Jackson, J.H. (1870). Digitalis with bromide of potassium in epilepsy. *Br. Med. J.*, **1**, 32
13. Gowers, W.R. (1881). *Epilepsy and other Chronic Convulsive Disorders: Their Causes, Symptoms and Treatment*. (London: Churchill)
14. Turner, W.A. (1907). *Epilepsy – a Study of the Idiopathic Disease*. (New York: Macmillan). (Reprinted, 1973, New York: Raven Press)
15. Rall, T.W. and Schleifer, L.S. (1985). Drugs effective in the treatment of epilepsy. In Goodman, L.S. and Gilman, A.G. (eds.) *Pharmacological Basis of Therapeutics*. 7th edn. (London: Macmillan)
16. Medical letter. (1970). Anticonvulsant drugs in idiopathic epilepsy. *Drugs and Therapy*, **12**, 53
17. Brodie, M.J. (1990). Status epilepticus in adults. *Lancet*, **336**, 36
18. Prior, P.F., Maclaine, G.N., Scott, D.F. and Laurance, B.M. (1972). Tonic status epilepticus precipitated by intravenous diazepam in a child with petit mal status. *Epilepsia*, **13**, 467
19. Tassinari, C.A., Gastaut, H., Dravet, C. and Roger, J. (1971). A paradoxical effect: status epilepticus induced by benzodiazepines, (Valium® and Mogadon®). *Electroencephalog. Clin. Neurophysiol.*, **31**, 629

10

Sodium valproate

The history of the discovery of sodium valproate is of considerable interest, not least because it remains a first-line drug, which is effective in all types of seizures including those of absence type – petit mal attacks in childhood[1]. The substance itself is different from other antiepileptic compounds, in not containing a nitrogen atom in the molecule. It was first synthesized as long ago as 1881, but only in 1962 were the therapeutic properties realized. Not long after this, a patent was taken out in France, where the work on the compound had been carried out.

The gap between the original synthesis and the discovery of the anticonvulsant actions was remarkable, being 80 years, indeed the longest interval for any marketed antiepileptic, in striking contrast to carbamazepine, where the time from first synthesis to the pharmacy shelves in most countries of the world was about 10 years. More recent discoveries, because of detailed requirements of testing before licensing (see Chapter 12), lead to a period which is often longer than that for carbamazepine. This is true, not only for antiepileptic drugs, but in addition for most other pharmaceuticals. A recent notable exception has been made by no lesser an authority than the FDA in relation to certain anti-AIDS compounds.

THE DISCOVERY

Valproic acid had been used widely for many years as a solvent for organic chemicals. In the year 1961, its true nature came to light when Mr Pierre Eymard was working under the supervision of Dr Meunier, at the laboratories of Berthier, located in Grenoble in France. During a screening procedure for antiepileptic activity in a number of compounds, he found that they all showed a strikingly similar, and unexpectedly marked, effect. Such overwhelming success was unusual at this routine screening stage. Then it was noted that the solvent, not the test compounds, had these beneficial effects. The first clinical trials were quickly underway by 1964. The results were quite clear-cut, and sodium valproate was first marketed in France in 1967. Other European countries soon followed suit, including the UK in 1974, the last European country where prescription was commenced. Like the US with carbamazepine, this was because of the stringent drug regulations.

Sodium valproate was discovered to be an anticonvulsant at the time when there was a particular interest in research of epilepsy in general, on both sides of the Atlantic. Not least in importance was the discovery of a new animal model (see below). One other particular advance was in the technology of blood level assessment. It was becoming more generally available. This method, coupled with the clear efficacy of sodium valproate for a wide spectrum of seizure disorders, led to an explosion of publications, estimated by 1991 to be in excess of 5000, whilst over a million individuals worldwide were by then receiving the compound. In spite of this wide experience and greater volume of research work, its mode of action remains unclear.

THE COST–BENEFITS EQUATION

Sodium valproate is a valuable drug in the treatment of epilepsy[2], with two-thirds of the patients showing a good response, that is, a 75–100% reduction in seizures[3]. Particularly valuable were the notable effects obtained in children with petit mal[4]. Patients who have drug resistant epilepsy, especially a combination of convulsions – tonic/clonic fits – and complex partial seizures, showed a less dramatic but useful change for the better[5]. From personal experience it seems the dosage may need to be high in this type of patient, though generally when sodium valproate is introduced, other anticonvulsants can be curtailed, so that toxic side-effects such as drowsiness, which accrue with large doses of different anticonvulsants given together, can be alleviated.

There are other considerations: first of all, the cost of a new drug such as sodium valproate is initially high, and indeed, it is still one of the more expensive antiepileptic compounds. Clearly the initial price to the consumer relates to the expense of research and development, including comprehensive toxicity studies in animals, and clinical trials in patients. This is likewise reflected, for example, in the cost of the newly introduced compounds, lamotrigine and vigabatrin. It seems certain that other antiepileptic drugs, even those yet to be discovered, are likely to be highly priced, a matter to be discussed in Chapter 12.

Toxicity

There are almost always new and unexpected unwanted effects with novel compounds. Sodium valproate was no exception. Though reports of problems continue to appear, they have not, quite rightly, prevented the drug from obtaining a prime place in the therapeutic armamentarium of the epileptologist. In connection with valproate there are three main concerns. The first relates to teratogenicity. As always, clear-cut answers to the patient's question, 'Will this drug affect my baby?' are not possible, not least because so often the patient, even nowadays, is receiving several other drugs at the same time. One particular condition that may arise from sodium valproate administration is neural tube defect. This often appears above the average in particular geographical areas, which may account for the early worrying reports. Sodium valproate is not necessarily contraindicated in those of child-bearing age, especially now that ultrasonic techniques may display tiny abnormalities of various types early enough in pregnancy to allow therapeutic intervention.

Hepatic toxicity is a well known complication of antiepileptic therapy, and presented a particular problem with sodium valproate before it was clearly recognized that the difficulty occurred almost exclusively in children. It could be noted early on by a clinician alert to the potential problem. The difficulty almost always arises when the drug is given in a regime of multiple antiepileptic drugs, the currently much despised polypharmacy.

The other complication, and this is not recognized for other antiepileptic compounds, is hair loss. Superficially, it may not seem to the prescribing physician to be unimportant in the cost–benefit equation, if the seizures are well controlled, but, particularly for teenagers of both sexes, it may be a reason for discontinuing the drug. Patients in this age group are notoriously unreliable. They will often not take 'no' for an answer, and may, if the physician does not comply, take the matter into their own hands! The reason for the unwanted side-effect remains unclear, but it is particularly important in this age group to be aware of the difficulties.

A NEW ANIMAL MODEL: THE BABOON

In parallel with the discovery of the antiepileptic action of sodium valproate, was the almost equally important development of a new animal model. To appreciate more fully the models previously discovered, it is important to understand the underlying processes in the central nervous system responsible for seizures, a matter considered further in Chapter 11. Here we will concentrate on the experimental paradigm presented by the baboon, and see how at least one aspect of antiepileptic action was clarified.

In the attempts to study the epileptic process fully, it becomes clear that the rodent model is inadequate, so primates need to be involved, in the first instance rhesus monkeys, and then the even more costly and rare baboons. They provide a prototype that is closest to the human syndromes of epilepsy, both in their pathophysiology, and also in their pharmacological responsiveness. First of all there is the use of the rhesus monkey with cortical implants of alumina gel[6]. This leads to a localized area of damage, and an epileptic focus as shown on the EEG, resulting in the development of motor seizures. There are other techniques too for producing lesions: heating, cooling and a variety of metals, as well as radioactive materials[7], though the results are largely similar.

In relation especially to sodium valproate, the baboon is more interesting. The animal lives in the wild in the African state of Senegal. It develops reflex epilepsy when exposed to intermittent flash stimulation provided by the stroboscope, widely used in the EEG laboratory[8]. This reflex epileptic disorder is one in which a specific stimulus regularly causes seizures. It is thus easily controllable and economic to use. In man, as well as stroboscopically delivered light (Figure 1), widely varying stimuli such as television, music and reading can lead to EEG changes and attacks in susceptible individuals, and can be tested systematically on each occasion the stimulus is presented.

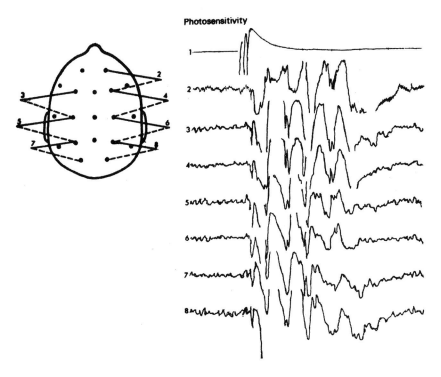

Photosensitivity

Figure 1 An example of the sudden change in EEG (channels 1–8) provoked by stroboscopic light stimulation. Channel 1 is the output from the monitoring photocell, and shows that only three flashes of light were required to induce high voltage generalized atypical spike and wave, not dissimilar to the other discharges seen either in the resting EEG, or evoked by photic stimulation, in petit mal epilepsy. (Reproduced from the author's *Understanding EEG*, Duckworth, 1976)

The alumina model in animals, in contrast, presents problems in that it is costly, because there may be a long interval, often many months, before seizures occur, and therefore the testing of a single drug, to see if the developed focus is suppressed, requires considerable periods of time. However, the photosensitive technique produces an instant response in susceptible animals. This was discovered interestingly quite by chance. It has the advantage that, with laboratory controlled intermittent light stimulation from the stroboscope, discharges in the EEG and attacks occur, as it were, 'to order'. The effect of anticonvulsant administration on these phenomena can be tested according to predetermined schedules, and repeated with a variety of compounds over a relatively short time span.

The curiosity of this animal observation is that only a proportion of baboons show it, and the prevalence changes from region to region of Senegal (Figure 2). The highest figure for responsiveness is for animals which come from the southern part, the Casamance area. Sodium valproate blocks the response regularly, as do other antiepileptic agents, such as phenobarbitone and benzodiazepines, for example, diazepam and clonazepam[9]. A high dosage of sodium valproate is required to produce the same effect.

The results of studies with sodium valproate and repeated photic stimulation of baboons parallel closely the blocking effect seen in man with the same paradigm[10]. The television set provides, for some susceptible patients, a similar provocative image and they have an abnormal response to the stroboscope (Figure 1). This is also shown by another small proportion of individuals who come to the EEG laboratory, certainly less than 5%[11]. This abnormality evoked in the EEG, and the seizures produced by viewing television, can be abolished by sodium valproate. There are comparable effects with barbiturates and benzodiazepines in line with antiepileptic actions found in animal paradigms with maximal electric shock and metrazol-induced seizures.

BASIC ASPECTS OF SEIZURE CAUSATION

Just how seizures are caused is a complex area. In essence, we can think of two fundamental processes which of course are not discrete, but for simplicity are often considered separately: firstly the neural and secondly the biochemical. The first was put forward by Hughlings Jackson[12], namely that epilepsy was a disorder of hyper-excitability of the nervous system. However, this does not, of course, take into account the great variety of clinical manifestations found in seizures, which because of their heterogeneity have for a long time defied rational classification, essential for accurate assessment of new antiepileptic agents. Now international definitions have been agreed, after many years of discussion, by committees of the International League Against Epilepsy, and published in various forms with modifications[13,14], and considerable deliberation[15].

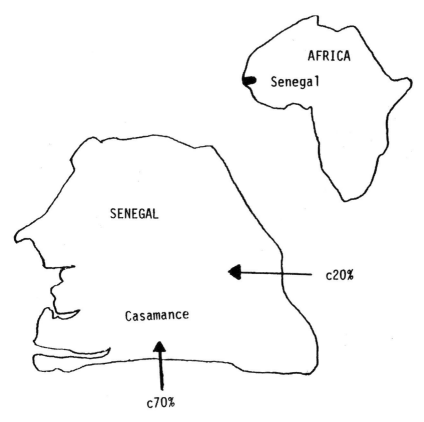

Figure 2 The marked discrepancy in response to intermittent photic stimulation between baboons from different areas of Senegal. (Redrawn from Naquet and Meldrum[8,9], with kind permission of authors and publishers)

Refining the Jackson definition, we now think of a focus of electrical discharge. This focus can arise on the basis of various pathological substrates, or, indeed, when excised at surgery for drug-resistant seizures, may show no pathological change whatsoever. It is therefore necessary to regard the fundamental disturbance as biochemical. The genesis of the focus is one aspect, but of crucial importance is the spread of electrical discharge. If this abnormality remains localized, there may be little or no clinical manifestation; if spread occurs, then depending on where the focus was located and to which area or areas it spreads, so the seizure will be focal or generalized subsequently.

EPILEPSY AND FIRE

Perhaps an analogy used previously[16] of a heath fire may be useful. A carelessly dropped match or cigarette end, we still do not know who is to blame, or what is responsible in the central nervous system, acts as a nidus for a possible subsequent conflagration. The breeze fans the embers to life, and depending on the amount of moisture in the surrounding heather, the focus may be extinguished or the vegetation may, with varying rates, smoulder and burst into flame – the focal, or when it spreads, the generalized seizure results.

The source of the still enigmatic electrical discharge in the primary focus, though uncertain, almost certainly relates to reduction in the inhibitory biochemical substances in the neuronal circuits. Small neurons with short axons, that are probably in part responsible, have via reverberatory loops, a local inhibitory effect. They are known to be particularly vulnerable to ischaemia, leading to hypoxic damage. In addition a great variety of compounds used therapeutically, varying from the frankly convulsant to such apparently innocuous groups of substances as antibiotics, may interfere with gamma-aminobutyric acid (GABA), the main inhibitory transmitter found in the brain. In experimental situations, electrical recordings may reveal neuronal bursts which are sudden, large and depolarizing, and lead to synchronous activity within wider neuronal networks. It is the spread of this excitatory potential – the so-called depolarizing shifts, that can be detected either by intracerebral or surface EEG recordings – which causes seizures. These are facilitated by, for example, changes in blood glucose concentration, pH and electrolyte composition of extracellular fluid.

This leads immediately to an equally simplistic view of how antiepileptic agents could or should act, namely suppress the focal neuronal discharge, and secondly reduce spread of excitation. It is this that brings about detonation of adjacent neurons and to the clinical seizure, if the process proceeds out of control.

CONCLUSION

Both the discovery of sodium valproate and the baboon model demonstrated once again that empirical factors are acting, chance, luck and serendipity were surprisingly at the forefront of progress.

Such a situation limits regular systematic progress. Perhaps this is changing – with a more rational approach. The final section of the book will hopefully show the way forward.

REFERENCES

1. Technical Manual. (1988). *Epilim, sodium valproate B.P.* (Manchester: Sanofi Pharmaceuticals)
2. Editorial. (1988). Sodium valproate. *Lancet*, **2**, 1229
3. Simon, D. and Penry, J.K. (1975). Sodium di-n-propylacetate (DPA) in the treatment of epilepsy. A review. *Epilepsia*, **16**, 549
4. Jeavons, P.M., Clarke, J.H. and Maheshwari, M.C. (1977). Treatment of generalised epilepsies in childhood and adolescence with sodium valproate (Epilim). *Dev. Med. Child Neurol.*, **19**, 9
5. Richens, A. and Ahmad, S. (1975). Controlled trial of sodium valproate in severe epilepsy. *Br. Med. J.*, **4**, 255
6. Ward, A.A. (1972). Topical convulsant metals. In Purpura, D.P., Penry, J.K., Tower, D.B., Woodbury, D.M. and Walters, R.D. (eds.) *Experimental Models of Epilepsy*. (New York: Raven Press)
7. Purpura, D.P., Penry, J.K., Tower, D.B., Woodbury, D.M. and Walter, R.D. (eds.) 1972. *Experimental Models of Epilepsy*. (New York: Raven Press)
8. Killam, K.F., Killam, E.K. and Naquet, R. (1966). Mise en évidence chez certain singes d'un syndrome photomyoclonique. *C. R. Acad. Sci. (Paris)*, **262**, 10
9. Meldrum, B.S. (1978). Photosensitive epilepsy in *Papio papio* as a model for drug studies. In Cobb, W.A. and van Duijn, H. (eds.) *Contemporary Clinical Neurophysiology*, (Suppl. 34). (Amsterdam: Elsevier)
10. Binnie, C.D., Kasteleijn-Nolst, T. and Korte, R. de. (1986). Photosensitivity as a model for acute anti-epileptic drug studies. *Electroencephalogr. Clin. Neurophysiol.*, **63**, 35
11. Jeavons, P.M. and Harding, G.F.A. (1975). Photosensitive epilepsy clinics. In *Developmental Medicine, No. 56*. (London: Heinemann)
12. Jackson, J.H. (1873). On the anatomical, physiological and pathological investigations of epilepsies. *West Riding Lunatic Asylum Med. Rep.*, **3**, 315
13. Gastaut, H. (1969). Clinical and electroencephalographical classification of epileptic seizures. International league against epilepsy. *Epilepsia*, **10** (Suppl.), S2
14. Gastaut, H. (1969). Classification of the epilepsies. *Epilepsia*, **10** (Suppl.), S14
15. Laidlaw, J. and Richens, A. (1982). Introduction in *A Textbook of Epilepsy*. (Edinburgh: Churchill)
16. Scott, D.F. (1973). *About Epilepsy*. (London: Duckworth)

11

Development of modern antiepileptic drugs in the 1990s

The past 20 years have been marked by considerable advance in the treatment of epilepsy. On the technological side there has been the widespread use of blood-level assessment of antiepileptic agents. This has been of considerable importance in the study of the biotransform of compounds, and the interaction between the various drugs, as well as the overall view of pharmacokinetics (Table 1). Coupled with this has been a marked swing from multiple drug administration to monotherapy.

NUMBER OF COMPOUNDS NOW AVAILABLE

There is another difference between the 1990s and several years ago. Look at the listing of commercially available antiepileptic drugs in the UK in the early 1990s; a surprisingly small number of different compounds are now available. Twenty years ago perhaps double that figure could be obtained on prescription; for example Coatsworth[1], in his review in 1971, listed 13 separate compounds. The change relates to the overall pattern of drug regulation. When legislation was first introduced, existing compounds were exempt: safety and efficacy testing was applied only to new pharmaceuticals being launched. Since then it has been necessary to produce evidence on toxicity and efficacy for compounds of long-standing. As a result, because of the cost of testing in a modern manner, many of these antiepileptic drugs have been deleted. It was obviously decided by individual companies that the profit likely to accrue by sale of these drugs in the foreseeable future was much less than the cost of laboratory and clinical trials.

Table 1   Stages in the pharmacodynamics of antiepileptic drugs

Dose given
Absorption occurs to a greater or lesser extent
Plasma levels rise, some drugs protein-bound, others free ⎫
Crosses the blood–brain barrier ⎬ metabolism
Brain tissue concentration rises ⎬ and excretion
Action at cell receptor sites ⎬ occur
Therapeutic effects and possible toxic actions ⎭

As long ago as 1971 Coatsworth[1] estimated that the cost of launching a new antiepileptic drug was in the order of millions of pounds. Taking into account inflation as well as the more rigorous testing schedules now carried out, this has multiplied several times since then. In recent years sodium valproate is the one new drug which could be regarded as successful, reaching a prime position with carbamazepine and phenytoin more quickly than expected. The estimates of the cost for testing and introduction, measured against the projected level of sales, were apparently in this case markedly discrepant, in favour of the pharmaceutical company.

Clearly the successful discovery of valproate, which can be attributed to serendipity, was the more remarkable because it was the first compound with proven efficacy for both absence and tonic/clonic seizures. As Porter[2] observes in relation to paradigms for testing the effect on these two sorts of fits, 'although these models are still used today and may represent the final pathway of many kinds of epileptic seizures, they tell us little about the mechanism of drug action and may not detect new and novel antiepileptic compounds'.

Such a disquiet is also felt by others who doubt that rational approaches will of necessity produce results, a subject to which attention is now devoted.

NEW DRUGS UNDER STUDY IN 1988

Already in the early 1980s the results of a systematic approach to discovery of new agents are available, and under clinical scrutiny. Indeed Meldrum and Porter[3] in their book *New Anticonvulsant Drugs*, with their contributors, indicated exciting possibilities. Now, only a

Table 2   The necessary characteristics of enzyme inhibitors as drugs

Pathway inhibition is likely to be therapeutic
No unwanted inhibition in other pathways
Compound has practical pharmacokinetics
Appropriate balance between benefit and risk, e.g. in toxicological studies
Extensive trial results satisfy regulatory authorities
Economically viable, i.e. can compete with other already available agents

few years later, two very serious horses in the race for success in the antiepileptic field, having burst from the starting gate, have fallen at one of the many hurdles and did not reach the finishing line – their names, progabide and zonisamide.

Nevertheless the search continues and in epilepsy, as in other fields, therapeutic attempts have been made to interrupt enzyme systems, so that improvement can be produced in various disorders.

There are criteria which enzyme inhibitors must fulfil to be effective (Table 2), whether they relate to the central nervous system or other parts of the body. In this category there are already over 30 compounds[4], autonomic drugs like phyostigmine, which inhibits choline esterase; cardiovascularly active compounds such as captropril, inhibiting the angiotensin converting enzyme (ACE); the antiviral agent, acyclovir, affecting DNA polymerase, and zidovudine (AZT) which acts on the enzyme reverse transcriptase. Levodopa is an important example of a compound used in the central nervous system.

It is just these searches for enzyme inhibitor systems that led to the discovery of vigabatrin (see below).

RATIONAL APPROACHES AND GAMMA-AMINOBUTYRIC ACID

Central to the epileptic process, as we saw in Chapter 10, is neuronal excitability. Updating the Hughlings Jackson hypothesis, Gastaut, a giant in the twentieth century's understanding of epilepsy, gave the definition as follows: 'a chronic brain disorder of various aetiologies characterized by recurrent seizures due to excessive discharge of cerebral neurons'.

Not only must the electrical potentials be considered, but also the biochemical substrate. Of crucial importance here is gamma-aminobutyric acid (GABA), known to be the main inhibitory transmitter in the human brain, being found in up to 40% of synapses. It was in 1950 that GABA was first identified as a unique chemical constituent of the brain, and its subsequent significance in the epileptic story resulted from detailed investigations by many different individuals, rather than the intervention of chance factors. Knowledge of this compound has been gained by animal studies: indeed, the importance of such investigations has been shown to be crucial in the development of our understanding of the central nervous system, which is closely guarded by a bony encasement (see Chapter 12). More is known about GABA than any other mammalian central inhibitory transmitter.

The first studies were carried out on crustaceans where there were peripheral inhibitory effects on motor fibres. Kravitz and co-workers[5] demonstrated that GABA was the only inhibitory amino acid involved. Subsequently, it has been shown that the release of GABA was correlated to the frequency of nerve stimulation. Recordings from muscle fibres indicated changes in the chloride ion which allowed GABA to be identified as a neurotransmitter.

The following features of GABA have been established. First, its synthesis is restricted almost entirely to the central nervous system, with only very small amounts in the peripheral nervous system or in organs. Secondly, its presence is restricted to those regions, because of the efficient blood–brain barrier across which it cannot pass. This of course as a corollary, means that oral medication, with GABA itself, for this reason alone will have little effect. Thirdly, GABA was noted to have a heterogeneous distribution, both in the brain and spinal cord, and fourthly, it was shown to have a turnover rate at least 10 and sometimes as much as 100, times greater than other transmitters present, for example, acetylcholine. Taken together, these factors established GABA's prime place as a neurotransmitter, important in epilepsy (see Chadwick[6] for review).

Inhibitory synapses have been demonstrated in various parts of the central nervous system, such as the cerebellum, the hippocampus and in the cerebral cortex. GABA mediates action through local interneurons and is also responsible for inhibition in the spinal cord. These pathways have been delineated by various workers using neurochemical and cytochemical methods, as well as by immuno-cytochemical techniques.

There are, however, several myths about GABA in relation to seizure control, including the following:

(1) Augmentation of GABA transmission acts only in specific, not all, brain regions.

(2) Elevation of GABA levels will always increase GABA in mediated transmission.

(3) Increased GABA transmission does always result in decreased brain excitability.

(4) GABA may interfere with seizure propagation but not necessarily initiation.

These have been forcefully made by Gale[7] on the basis of animal experimentation, though here one could argue that the particular animal model used might not be totally relevant to man. Nevertheless the views of Gale are as important as they are provocative. They show at the very least, if we needed to be reminded, that the central nervous system is a highly complex network and the apparently rational attempts to unravel isolated systems may be fraught with great problems.

THE CHEMISTRY OF GABA

The next stage was to determine how GABA was metabolized, and the pathways for breakdown. This would then indicate to the pharmaceutical chemists where they might find critical points in metabolic pathways suitable for interruption. So possibly at last the discovery of anticonvulsant substances might become a process of intellect and ingenuity in synthetic chemistry, rather than the hap-hazard process by which antiepileptic drugs have been discovered previously.

GABA is formed by the action of the enzyme, glutamic acid decarboxylase (GAD), for which glutamic acid is a substrate and the main provider of the inhibitor (Table 3). This is confirmed by the effects of convulsant compounds, such as bicuculine, picrotoxin and

Table 3 Stages in metabolism of gamma-aminobutyric acid (GABA)

Synthesized by glutamic acid decarboxylase (GAD) in presynaptic nerve
    terminals, from glutamic acid
Released during neurotransmission
Taken up by receptors and glial cells
Opens neighbouring calcium channels
Thus electrically stabilizes the postsynaptic membrane
Re-enters presynaptic nerve terminals
Or is destroyed by GABA amino-transferase (GABA-T)

metrazol, all of which are selective antagonists of GABA. Interestingly, as we have already mentioned (Chapter 9), there is a close
relationship between binding sites of GABA and those for benzodiazepine compounds, and interaction occurs. However, the matter is
not straightforward, since there appear to be two types of receptor for
GABA that have been labelled A and B.

The breakdown of GABA proceeds, and this is an important
observation, through a reversible reaction which is brought about by
the enzyme GABA-transaminase, abbreviated to GABA-T. This
enzyme is not found exclusively in the neurons, but also in the glial
cells. Fortunately these enzyme systems can be studied in mammalian
brain slices, rather than requiring an intact animal. Such methods
obviously make investigations easier and quicker, but of course the
findings do have to be applied, not only in mammalian species, but
finally in man. This clearly represents a hurdle to be jumped,
involving efficacy studies of compounds and evidence concerning
relative toxicity.

Other amino acids are of importance; glycine is the building brick
for GABA, but is not itself a potent agent. In contrast, glutamate and
aspartate, which are found in very high concentrations in the brain,
have extremely powerful excitatory effects on neurons. Clearly study
of these compounds, and how they are broken down, is of major
importance for understanding the brain chemistry of seizure
disorders. The level of excitability is arrived at by the solution of an
equation in which the amino acids and their appropriate enzymes are
all factors.

TARGETS FOR THE CHEMISTS

Taking a general view of the complex series of *in vivo* biochemical reactions involving GABA, it can be appreciated that to maximize inhibition, either the production must be increased or the breakdown retarded. The former has not yet been achieved, but attempts at the latter course of action have proved successful. The fact that the chemistry of GABA is much more involved that this simplistic view is shown by the inability, at least so far, to determine exactly the mechanism of the action of a compound such as sodium valproate. However, taking the possible models of chemistry suggested above, biochemists have been able to synthesize potential anticonvulsants.

PROGABIDE

GABA itself does not cross the blood–brain barrier, but the precursor progabide, or pro-drug, to use the accurate pharmacological terminology, does do just that, entering the CNS and being metabolized by GABA. At an experimental level[8], it has been pointed out that progabide has a wide range of anticonvulsant actions, and a potency comparable with major anticonvulsant drugs in current use, having also the advantage of a beneficial effect on mood and behaviour in children. However, establishing its place in the therapeutic armamentarium remains to be achieved. This, as in many other instances, involves drug evaluation in efficacy studies along with the careful reporting of side-effects. Progabide apparently leads to a disturbance of hepatic enzymes, not an uncommon problem with new drugs. They are invariably used as an addition to the other antiepileptic drugs that the chronic patient is receiving. Then naturally there is difficulty in determining whether an observed toxicity, such as disturbance of liver enzymes, relates directly to the drug under study, or to other compounds given simultaneously, or whether it is in fact linked to the total 'load' of the antiepileptic drugs which is now larger than before. This load factor is well known to be important in relation to teratogenicity.

A meta-analysis[8] showed benefit in about 35% of patients, also observed by other authors. However, the final place of the compound in therapy remains very uncertain.

VIGABATRIN

In the 1970s the mechanism of action of valproate was thought to be via GABA-T inhibition and the search for a better GABA-T blocker was begun by Merrell Dow's chemists. They were successful, but the compound they obtained had quite different characteristics from those of valproate.

Catabolism of GABA takes place by means of GABA-T. The work by Merrell Dow scientists involved a new concept. In simple terms, the GABA-T enzyme cannot distinguish between the naturally occurring substance on which it acts, and an enzyme-activated inhibitor chemical (Figure 1). An irreversible bond is established between the GABA-T and this enzyme-activated inhibitor, and as a result the GABA-T is rendered permanently inactive. The advantage of this approach is twofold. Firstly, there is a high degree of selectivity, and secondly, the inhibition is irreversible with resulting long duration of action, which is only overcome by the body's manufacturing new enzymes. This may take days to accomplish.

Two substances with the requirements were synthesized. The first, an acetylenic derivative, proved to be less specific than had been hoped. Research continued on the second, namely gamma-vinyl GABA – vigabatrin, which was more selective. This is now available for treatment of patients. The added advantage of this drug is the lack of other effects on substances involved in the GABA breakdown[9].

Of course various animal models have been employed in the testing of vigabatrin. It is active against maximal electroshock models, and the reflex seizures induced by auditory stimuli. Interestingly vigabatrin is also effective in controlling the manifestations of photic stimulation in baboons[10], a feature of the action of sodium valproate (see Chapter 10).

NEW DRUGS, NOVEL NEUROTOXICITY

Porter[2] pertinently observes, 'as we cleverly devise new neuro-active drugs, we therefore encounter novel forms of neurotoxicity, some of which will undoubtedly prove to be benign neuropathological curiosities, whilst others may be genuinely troublesome'. This was the situation in relation to vigabatrin. The real problem is attempting

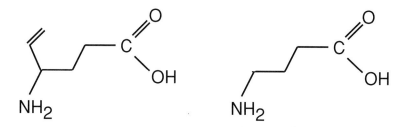

Figure 1 Similarity of the active chemical structure of vigabatrin (left) and gamma-aminobutyric acid (GABA) (right), indicating why the former presents a 'suicidal' substrate for the enzyme GABA amino transferase, which is responsible for the degradation of GABA[2]

to decide which of the findings reported by patients or observed in the animal studies are truly toxic and which not. Clearly the fate of many important and potentially major new drug discoveries hangs in the balance.

In the course of studies on vigabatrin, small lesions were discovered in the brains of animals used for chronic toxicity testing. These lesions appeared to be due to splitting of the myelin sheath. Myelin itself can be regarded as the main insulator of the nervous pathways and therefore potentially of prime importance. These changes occurred in a variety of species, but were noted to disappear when the drug was withdrawn. Nevertheless, it was important to decide whether the change observed in animals was benign and therefore of little consequence, or could have occurred in man with possibly devastating effects.

A number of points had to be taken into account in this context. Was there any lack of development of myelin? This was not the case. Next, when long-term exposure studies were carried out it was found that the lesions did not progress; also on the positive side was the reversal of the drug action after discontinuation. Also, when vigabatrin was given, no neurophysiological changes were found in man. Further, when part of the brain from patients receiving vigabatrin was removed during surgical treatment of the epilepsy, because drug therapy was ineffective, no neurochemical or neuropathological changes were observed. The same is true of autopsy specimens from patients who unfortunately died, either as a result of epilepsy or other causes. Consequent on these observations, development of the drug and use in humans proceeded.

By 1990 the compound had satisfied the drug regulatory authorities in the UK, with the proviso that vigabatrin could only be used in those patients who had been shown to be previously drug-resistant. Indeed for this inauspicious group it transpired that half the patients showed a 50% reduction in attacks or even better results[11]. It has also been approved for clinical use in virtually every country in Europe.

LAMOTRIGINE

Another compound with a totally new structure in relation to antiepileptic action has been developed by another company, Wellcome. It is currently under clinical trial to prove efficacy as monotherapy and has, in 1991, been given a licence for use in chronic patients. The site of action of lamotrigine is quite different from that of vigabatrin.

The discovery of lamotrigine

The lamotrigine saga began many years ago with the observation of low serum folates in some patients with epilepsy, which when corrected by folic acid supplements led to a worsening of the seizures[12]. Researchers as a result looked for antifolate compounds which might be antiepileptic and could be used in treatment. One of these was lamotrigine and this was selected for development. However, it emerged that its mode of action is not in relation to folate, but rather that it interferes with glutamate transmission! Glutamate is in the excitatory part of the GABA 'equation' and of crucial importance[13].

The final place of lamotrigine in treatment is uncertain but on the positive side, apart from skin rashes, there are few adverse side-effects. The dose level of lamotrigine has to be adjusted because of interaction with enzyme-inhibiting antiepileptic drugs as well as with valproate. As with other new pharmaceuticals the high price to the prescriber will be a factor to be considered, particularly in under-developed countries.

GABAPENTIN

Another novel drug, gabapentin, has a chemical formula related to the structure, as its name implies, of GABA. It was synthesized to mimic the action of this compound and cross the blood–brain barrier freely. However, the original supposition was not supported in animal studies of pharmacology or electrophysiology. These investigations showed that, although the compound is active in controlling the seizures induced both chemically and electrically, it does not change the postsynaptic GABA or glutamate responses. Further, there is no suppression of spontaneous neural activity or blockade of high frequency sustained action potentials which are akin to seizure discharges. In these respects it contrasts with first-line drugs – phenytoin, carbamazepine and valproate.

On the positive side, gabapentin is relatively free of adverse effects, while on the negative side there is a suggestion of possible carcinogenicity. This finding has recently emerged and requires further investigation. Because of its low overall toxicity, its place in the armamentarium of epileptologists seems assured, but, as with new compounds in the field, compared with established drugs, gabapentin is rather costly.

There are yet more substances under study (see Table 3, Chapter 12), and other animal models have been developed in this context, the paradigm which has been labelled 'kindling' being the most recent.

KINDLING

The very name 'kindling' is evocative, with its obvious reference to lighting a fire. This analogy was used previously (see Chapter 10) in relation to the initiation and propagation of the individual seizure. Here the notion is extended in terms of the time base, and deals with not just the start of a single attack, but the genesis of the whole complex process, particularly the seizure threshold.

Kindling was first described in rats[14], but has been extended to other animal species. The process is dependent on regular, often daily, intermittent electrical stimulation to susceptible brain areas, notably the amygdala and hippocampus. The level of shock chosen is below that which would provoke a seizure there and then. After repeated stimuli at the same level, seizures are provoked, and at that stage with even smaller currents, fits are observed.

The next stage is the development of spontaneous seizures, that is, those which happen without a provoking electrical stimulus. It has been likened to the spontaneous seizures, usually convulsions, that occur in previously non-epileptic psychiatric patients who require repeated courses of electroconvulsive therapy for either depressive or schizophrenic illness, and apparently as a result develop seizures[15]. The model has also been likened to that in man of the appearance of the so-called mirror focus. Here the source of electrical stimulation is in the brain already, for example in one temporal lobe. Due to a pathological process, electrical firing is occurring actively, and the potentials impinge via connecting neurons to the homologous region on the other side. This, after a latent period of the order of years, begins spontaneously, not only to discharge, but also to provoke clinical attacks.

The other crucial aspect in relation to therapy is the abolition of amygdala-kindled seizures. It can be achieved in various ways, for example, by focal injection into the substantia nigra. Vigabatrin is one substance, administered in this way, that has such an effect[16]. Further, when a seizure occurs as a result of the spread of electrical discharge in the limbic, hippocampal or basal ganglionic structures, such as the substantia nigra, the change can be visualized and, indeed, quantified in terms of cerebral blood flow and the utilization of the essential brain nutrient, glucose[17].

THE VALUE OF KINDLING

Kindling is an excellent model, since it produces a long-lasting seizure susceptibility which is sufficient to produce recurrent, spontaneous electrical seizures. They may initially be focal in type and become secondarily generalized. The spontaneous attacks in the amygdala-kindled cat, perhaps surprisingly, show exactly the pattern found in human epilepsy, in terms of electrical and clinical events seen before, during and after the seizure, namely the pre-ictal, ictal and postictal manifestations[18]. We therefore have a valid model for epilepsy[19]. It has indeed proved to be particularly useful in elucidating the chemistry of GABA and other central nervous system substances which are either excitatory or inhibitory in effect, providing a rational basis for improved therapeutic approaches to intractable epilepsy.

This is especially emphasized by the actions that different antiepileptic drugs have on the kindling process[19]. Phenobarbitone, carbamazepine and valproate suppress amygdala-kindled seizures and, more importantly, in doses that have a minimal behavioural toxic effect. The same is true of benzodiazepines, such as diazepam. This contrasts with succinamides like ethosuximide, which act specifically on petit mal, and are ineffective in this particular model.

THE PROPHYLACTIC USE OF ANTIEPILEPTICS

Kindling has potentially a direct relevance in a particular clinical situation which is still, like so many aspects of the understanding and treatment of seizure disorders, controversial, namely the prophylactic use of anticonvulsant agents in populations who have a risk, often a high risk, of developing seizures as a complication of a basic disorder. Numerically the most important of these is head injury; in developed countries road traffic accidents are of prime importance. Another group of patients are those who have neurosurgical procedures requiring craniotomy, for example, in the treatment of cerebral neoplasms or vascular anomalies, such as aneurysms and arterial malformations, procedures which also carry a risk of subsequent epilepsy. A further category of importance is that of children who develop, in the absence of any neurosurgical procedure, febrile seizures.

The kindling model, which shows effects which differ from antiepileptic agent to agent, is notable in respect to prophylaxis. Phenobarbitone, for example, has this action par excellence, but has troublesome side-effects, whilst carbamazepine is non-prophylactic. Clinical studies have shown that medication given to high-risk patients within hours of head injury, and even if only continued for 3 months, may have a long-lasting protective action against developing a seizure disorder[20]. Evidence was put forward in this matter in relation to non-traumatic conditions, for example, following aneurysm surgery[21,22], and information continues to accrue on the subject, but a consensus view remains to be established[23].

When and why do seizures cease?

There are two aspects to the cessation of seizures. First, why does the individual seizure stop, and second, what needs to be done about antiepileptic medication if there have been no atttacks for several years.

The individual seizure is believed to be caused by the local aggregation of excitatory transmitters, glutamate and possibly aspartate, arising as the result of electrical activity involving reverberatory neuronal circuits. The inhibitory GABA is overwhelmed. The seizure discharge thus initiated spreads, and a fit results. Cessation is probably principally achieved by a build up of GABA, but this is not the whole story, because recently opioids, known to be produced in the brain, may also play an inhibiting role in terminating a seizure[25]. This remains to be proven. However, in patients who have one absence, petit mal, attack after another, a sequence almost amounting to a form of status epilepticus, but less severe than that of the convulsive type, endogenous opioids are involved in cessation[26]. These observations suggest a possible new strategy in the search for antiepileptic medication[26].

When to discontinue antiepileptic drugs

In a proportion of patients medication controls seizures completely. Just what proportion depends on the population under study. The response to treatment can roughly be divided in thirds, one third showing a very good or excellent benefit, another third responding with a significant reduction in attacks, while the remainder consist of those with little response, and those with continuing frequent or even worsening seizures. It is in this group that the new drugs are crucial, with advances as they emerge from the pharmaceutical industry.

However, for very fortunate individuals who are fit-free, a decision has to be made as to when to reduce and discontinue the antiepileptic medication. The decision depends on a detailed consideration as to whether a relapse would be serious. This could, for example, present a problem in the work place, or lead to loss of a driving licence. Discussion between physician and patient is clearly important in this situation, when the benefit of stopping the drugs is weighed against the cost of relapse. Generally, reduction of medication, never sudden cessation, which can precipitate status epilepticus, is not contemplated, until the patient is free of attacks for at least two years. This is an area of controversy, and one where research is currently in progress. Discussion is outside the scope of the text, and reviews should be consulted, particularly as there may be differences in policy for adults [27,28], compared with children [29].

In conclusion, it is clear that many problems still exist regarding the treatment of epilepsy and the drugs currently available and being developed. What the future holds is of great potential, and is our concern in the next and final chapter.

REFERENCES

1.   Coatsworth, J.J. (1971). Studies on the clinical efficacy of marketed anti-epileptic drugs. *NINDS Monograph, No. 12.* (Bethesda, Maryland: US Dept. of Health, Education and Welfare)
2.   Porter, R.J. (1990). New anti-epileptic agents; strategies of drug development. *Lancet*, **336**, 423
3.   Meldrum, B.S. and Porter, R.J. (eds.) (1986). *New Anticonvulsant Drugs.* (London: John Libbey)
4.   Crout, R.J. (1990). Enzyme inhibitors as drugs. In *Enzymes as Targets for Drug Design.* (New York: Academic Press)
5.   Kravitz, E.A., Kuffler, S.W. and Potter, D.D. (1963). Gamma-amino butyric acid and other blocking compounds in crustacea. *J. Neurophysiol.*, **26**, 739
6.   Chadwick, D.W. (1990). New therapeutic horizons in epilepsy. In Kennard, C. (ed.) *Recent Advances in Clinical Neurology, No. 6.* (Edinburgh, London: Churchill Livingstone)
7.   Gale, K. (1989). GABA in epilepsy: the pharmacological basis. *Epilepsia*, **32** (Suppl. 3) (New York: Raven)
8.   Morselli, P.L., Bartholini, G. and Lloyd, K.G. (1986). Progabide. In Meldrum, B.S. and Porter, R.G. (eds.) *New Anticonvulsant Drugs.* (London: John Libbey)
9.   Symposium (1990). *Vigabatrin: a new anti-epileptic agent.* (Oxford: Medicare Group (UK) Ltd.)
10. Meldrum, B.S. and Horton, R. (1978). Blockage of epileptic responses in the photosensitive baboon, *Papio papio*, by two irreversible inhibitors of GABA transaminase γ-acetylenic GABA (4-amino-hex-5-enone acid) and γ-vinyl GABA. *Psychopharmacology*, **59**, 47
11. Brodie, M.J. and Porter, R.J. (1990). New and potential anticonvulsants. *Lancet*, **336**, 27
12. Reynolds *et al.* (1966). Anticonvulsant therapy, megaloblastic haemopoiesis and folic acid metabolism. *Q. J. Med.*, **35**, 521

13. Brodie, M.J. and Porter, R.G. (1990). New and potential anticonvulsants. *Lancet*, **336**, 27

14. Goddard, G.V., McIntyre, D.C. and Leech, C.K. (1969). A permanent change in brain function resulting from daily electrical stimulation. *Exp. Neurol.*, **25**, 295

15. Naoi, T. (1959). Electroencephalographic study on the electric convulsive treatment. *Psychiatr. Neurol. (Jpn.)*, **61**, 871

16. McNamara, J.O., Galloway, M.T., Rigsbee, L.C. and Shin, C. (1984). Evidence implicating the substantia nigra in the regulation of kindled seizure threshold. *J. Neurosci.*, **4**, 2410

17. Ueno, H., Yamashita, Y. and Caveness, W.F. (1975). Regional cerebral blood flow in focal epileptiform seizures in the monkey. *Exp. Neurol.*, **47**, 81

18. Wada, J.A., Sato, M. and Corcoran, M.E. (1974). Persistent seizure susceptibility and recurrent spontaneous seizures in kindled cats. *Epilepsia*, **15**, 465

19. Sato, M., Racine, R.J. and McIntyre, D.C. (1990). Kindling: basic mechanisms and clinical validity. *Electroencephalogr. Clin. Neurophysiol.*, **76**, 459

20. Young, B., Rapp, R., Brooks, W.H. and Madnuss, W. (1979). Post-traumatic epilepsy prophylaxis. *Epilepsia*, **20**, 671

21. Cabral, R., King, T.T. and Scott, D.F. (1976). Incidence of postoperative epilepsy after a transtentorial approach to acoustic nerve tumours. *J. Neurol. Neurosurg. Psychiatr.*, **39**, 663

22. Cabral, R., King, T.T. and Scott, D.F. (1976). Epilepsy after two different approaches to the treatment of ruptured intracranial aneurysm. *J. Neurol. Neurosurg. Psychiatr.*, **39**, 666

23. Jennett, B. (1982). Post-traumatic epilepsy. In Laidlaw, J. and Richens, A. (eds.) *A Textbook of Epilepsy*. (Edinburgh: Churchill Livingstone)

24. Willmore, L.J. (1992). Post-traumatic epilepsy – mechanism and prevention. In Pedley, T.A. and Meldrum, B.S. (eds.) *Recent Advances in Epilepsy*. (Edinburgh: Churchill Livingstone)

25. Tortella, F.C. (1988). Endogenous opioid peptides and epilepsy: quieting the seizing brain. *TIPS*, **9**, 366–72

26. Duncan, J.S., Bartenstein, P.A., Fish, D.R., Frackowiak, R.S.J. and Brooks, D.J. (1991). Investigation of generalised absence seizures using [11]C. d. prenorphine and positron emission tomography. *J. Cereb. Blood Flow Metab.*, **11** (Suppl. 2), 414

27. Overweg, J. (1985). *Withdrawal of Antiepileptic Drugs in Seizure-free Adult Patients; Prediction of Outcome*. (Amsterdam: Rodopi)

28. Chadwick, D. (1990). Diagnosis of epilepsy. *Lancet*, **336**, 15

29. Keränen, T. (1990). Discontinuation of antiepileptic drugs. In Sillanpää, M., Johannessen, S.I. and Blemow, G.D. (eds.) *Paediatric Epilepsy*. (Petersfield: M. Wrightson Biochemical Publications Ltd.)

12

The future

There are many aspects of epilepsy that have not been covered in the preceding chapters because discovery and the use of specific antiepileptic agents have no direct relevance. However, in order that the reader is aware of the author's overall interests, two examples of specific matters that emerged in 1 week at a clinic for patients with intractable seizure disorders are now recalled.

One was the death of a 29-year-old man in a single seizure – not status epilepticus – because it was witnessed by his wife, and the second, the prosecution of an 18-year-old woman who had apparently taken something from a shop following a seizure. These are just two incidents among many that could be cited, in which help is required from the physician and other care-workers. It is important that the reader knows that there are various problems in the treatment of epilepsy; even so control of seizures with drugs can often be of greatest significance.

TO THE FUTURE

What then is the future for research? It is to discover new antiepileptic agents. Clearly, to continue a logical programme using the current knowledge of brain biochemistry is essential. This involves animal work prior to studies in human volunteers, later on patients with intractable seizures. A broad and varied range of clinical investigation must be carried out, as put forward by Cereghino and Penry[1] almost 20 years ago. No-one can deny that accurate diagnosis of syndromes and baseline data on seizure frequency is absolutely essential for assessment. This is similar to the problems encountered for such chronic attacks as migraine and angina. There are other possible avenues for investigation suggested by analogy, on the basis of recent research into chronic disorders, including those affecting the nervous system.

All these methods may, at least initially, weigh heavily on the findings of new animal models. There is a current general concern on ethical matters in relation to this research, and the exploration for new non-animal methods, which could be employed in screening and would be quicker and therefore cheaper, is essential.

HISTORY OF ANIMAL RESEARCH

First of all, let us consider the history of the use of animals in medicine. This has yielded great advancement in knowledge as well as in treatment. Researchers in medical matters have used animals for thousands of years. There is an ancient Greek reference, by Alcmaeon of Croton dated about 500 BC, which showed that blindness occurred if the optic nerve in a dog was severed. A little later in the Hippocratic writings it is recorded that coloured water was fed to a pig and its path traced after dissection of the animal.

In the 17th century, schools of anatomy made big strides forward by studies on animals and dissection of cadavers. The value of animal experimentation can be supported by the list of discoveries made in this way: the lymphatic system was defined by Aselli in 1627, the circulation of the blood by Harvey in 1628, and the function of the lungs by Robert Hook in 1663. Recently vivisection experiments have been directed towards cures for human kidney disease, coronary artery disease, asthma, leukaemia, diabetes, rheumatism and arthritis as well as innumerable infections. Of particular importance recently have been discoveries in relation to antiviral agents, for example the treatment of the formerly universally fatal herpes simplex encephalitis.

Many people accept the use of rodents, but are more upset by experiments on dogs, horses and monkeys. However, in studies directed to neurological disorders such as parkinsonism it is necessary to use primates, as in AIDS research. However, these studies represent less than 1% of all the research carried out; 85% is performed on mice, rats, guinea pigs, birds (mainly chickens) and some on rabbits.

THE SCIENTIST VERSUS THE ANTIVIVISECTIONIST

Many claims made by animal activists are totally inaccurate, or as Sir Walter Bodmer, Director of the Imperial Cancer Research Fund in the UK, says, they are simply wrong. Here are some examples: it is stated that animal experiments have done nothing to help in prevention of disease. Further that the investigations carried out on animals are irrelevant to humans. They, it is suggested, could be replaced by experiments on tissue cultures and by use of computer simulation; and finally the scientists are unwilling to use alternatives. All these views are quite misguided and have been countered by a declaration signed by many Nobel Prize winners as well as other scientists.

PARALLELS WITH CANCER RESEARCH

For 35 years US scientists working in the National Cancer Institute have been using mice in screening programmes. More than 400 000 chemicals have been injected into leukaemic mice. The hope was to find chemotherapeutic agents that would help not only to treat but to solve the riddles of malignant disease. All these investigations have produced only 36 licensed drugs, most of them effective against leukaemia but with only a modest value in other forms of cancer. Perhaps, therefore, the wrong screening device has been used? This was the observation of one of the senior members of the programme.

Such a question could also be asked about the methods used for the preliminary testing of antiepileptic agents, but what else could be used in such a screening programme? The alternatives, which are now being explored both for malignant disease and epilepsy but also for many chronic disorders, have included an arsenal of automated devices and computers, to test potential drugs on tissue cultures taken from humans, but grown in the laboratory. Such a process enabled scientists in a cancer programme to check such a staggering number as more than 300 different substances every week. To their surprise they found that drugs which passed the earlier mice testing were not discarded by the newer, sophisticated process, suggesting that mouse testing alone may lead to the rejection of potentially valuable compounds. Naturally there still has to be the ultimate test of efficacy in humans and regulation of this process (see Table 1). Some

159

Table 1   Main aspects of drug regulation (based on Mann[2])

The pharmaceutical industry requires independent regulation, in the public
   interest
The regulatory authority supervises safety, quality and efficacy of new
   products
Drug regulation is science-based, free from political or economic
   considerations
Regulatory process seen to be professional and scientific, medically based
   within and outside pharmaceutical industry
Granting a product licence based on safety, etc. at time of submission, i.e.
   limited in numbers of patients and follow-up duration
Post-marketing surveillance essential

observations on discoveries in medicine came from Bishop who with
Harold Varmus received a Nobel Prize in 1989 for their innovative
studies on cancer.

BACKGROUND TO NEW FINDINGS

Bishop put it as follows: 'I have learned that there is no single path to
creativity, not even within the stern halls of science ... we are
constrained not only by the necessary discipline of rigour but by the
limits of our imagination and our intellectual courage'[3].

He continues by explaining that discovery takes several forms.
First of all there is its mundane aspect which is nevertheless
important. He regards it as a 'groping stage' and this is followed by
the search for proof of the reality of the earlier procedures. He also
points out that looking back, there are among the discoveries many
missed opportunities, and failures to recognize the importance of a
particular observation.

Chance appeared to be operating in relation to the work of Bishop
and Varmus. They came together, with various skills, to posts in the
same place in California and worked together, taking as their starting
point viral studies in relation to cancerous growth. It is recollected as
follows 'we just staggered into it'. However, their discoveries spanned
6 years of intense study and they recalled that there was no moment
of sudden recognition of an important discovery. Their field was the
chemistry of the retrovirus in cancer research. One might have

expected firm statements on such a rational application of a new programme, but to our surprise the expert invokes 'casino factors' saying 'it is a high-risk venture, but it's a gamble worth taking', and hoping for results, 'all it will take is one smashing winner. Then everyone will say it was worth it'. As for cancer, so in epilepsy, we await the wonder drug or other solutions.

DISCOVERY OF ANTIBIOTICS

In the history of antibiotics the occurrence of a happy accident in 1928 resulted in the discovery of penicillin by Alexander Fleming (1881–1955). The culture plate was left exposed when he was on holiday and had not, as should have happened, been disinfected by the laboratory assistant before Fleming returned. Nevertheless, it required his appreciation of the results to clinch the finding that penicillin had inhibited bacterial growth. He was awarded the Nobel Prize for medicine in 1945 with the two brilliant chemists, Florey and Chain, who perfected the method for the manufacture of the compound in quantity. Hence it was a combination of chance and luck and, most important, serendipity.

What happens nowadays? In spite of the fact that most drugs are carefully mapped out by computer in the pharmacological laboratory, it is said that researchers from the company, Glaxo, still collect soil samples when holidaying abroad, because in the past chance findings from these have proved the source of valuable antibiotics[4]. Here is an age when we pride ourselves on a rational approach, yet we still like to invoke chance factors, even having a flutter on a race or a bet on the football pools, feeling we deserve to make a fortune, whilst knowing that the odds against us for such an outcome are phenomenal.

THE EMPIRICAL VERSUS THEORETICAL APPROACH

In the course of this book it has been emphasized that discovery of anticonvulsant drugs not only concerned the synthesis of compounds, but also the means of their testing. Animal models were regarded as of crucial importance exemplified in the work of Putnam and Merritt[5], and as time passed more models were added to the armamentarium of the screening process available to the pharmaceutical chemists.

However, it may be argued that those drugs discovered serendipitously or with a happy mixture of luck and chance in addition – the casino factors – were particularly potent and did not need models to test them on, or clinical trials to assess them by. Digitalis is an example of this. It has stood the test of time and if an attempt had been made to introduce the drug today, through the various hoops of toxicity testing and clinical trials, it is possible that digitalis would not in fact be available as perhaps the most potent drug available to cardiologists.

Let us consider the situation with streptomycin in the treatment of tuberculous meningitis. The condition had been, if not fatal, almost invariably leading to serious neurological morbidity. Immediately after streptomycin was introduced the situation was completely reversed and no clinical trial was necessary to prove the value of the compound.

The cynic could argue that any drug that requires a clinical trial must by its nature have not shown itself in open studies to have any major effect, and therefore almost by definition, is not a particularly potent agent. This then turns on its head the thesis that change from an empirical to a rational approach in the development of therapeutic agents is likely to be successful!

COST OF RESEARCH

Another aspect concerns the cost of research programmes, considerable not least because they are time consuming. Research and development costs are commonly 10–15% of the annual sales of pharmaceutical companies, and therefore enormous (see Table 2). This is much more than for the so-called high tech industries such as telecommunications and electronics. The drug sector in many countries is among the biggest civilian employer of scientists and technicians.

Another problem is that over the past 10 years the safety rules have become more onerous, not unnaturally driven by public scares over such drugs as thalidomide and Opren®. They have pushed up research and development costs, but in a sense it is more worrying that only a quarter of the bill is accounted for by pure research, the rest covers the development needed to drive new products through the regulatory mechanisms. It has lengthened the time it takes to get a

Table 2 The world's largest drug companies and their sales in billions of dollars[6]

Company	Sales	Company	Sales
Merck (US)	5.02	Takeda (Japan)	2.43
Bristol Myers/Squibb (US)	3.78	American Home (US)	2.35
Glaxo (UK)	3.62	Pfizer (US)	2.33
Smith Kline Beecham (UK)	3.61	Sandoz (Switzerland)	2.31
Ciba-Geigy (Switzerland)	2.91	Eli Lilly (US)	2.27
Hoechst (Germany)	2.80		

new formulation on sale. The time for approval for a new drug has leapt from just a few years to a figure now nearer 12 years[6]. There are several stages in drug regulation which are clearly necessary and require not only considerable work but time to complete (Table 1).

DISCOVERING THE NEW AND RE-TESTING THE OLD

Problems arise in relation to drug development and the patent laws. At the present time 20 years is allowed after the application for patenting of a new drug, but half or more of this time may in fact be used in various forms of testing. So certain drugs such as antiepileptic compounds, which have usually only that single use and therefore a relatively small population to which they can be prescribed, are not given priority in drug firm economics. The pressure to advance and find new drugs is much less here, than for blood-lipid lowering agents, where the drug has also to be given chronically but the patient population is much larger – obviously a much better investment for a pharmaceutical firm. Perhaps as Grattini[7] suggests the patent should last for 30 years. This would increase the 'pay-back' for successful drugs and provide the resources for further research and development.

There is another matter of consequence. Many thousands of chemicals synthesized in the past were developed with a particular indication in mind. If the drug did not seem to be efficacious in this respect, its patent would expire and no further action could be taken.

However, there are nowadays many screening tests available which were not envisaged when chemicals were synthesized earlier. These include new chemical mediators, growth factors, secondary messengers, enzymes and so on, which could be used for targets of drug action. If there was a facility for re-patenting the compound then there would be an impetus to retest many compounds currently 'on the shelf'. There is an example of this in epilepsy therapy. In the 1930s when Putnam was looking into the possibility of the antiepileptic action of diphenyl compounds he was able, from the company Parke Davis, to obtain samples of compounds which had been synthesized almost 20 years before and had remained on the shelf, because at that stage they were shown not to have an hypnotic action, the purpose of their synthesis.

NEURAL GRAFTING

Another possible approach in therapy is neural grafting, or cellular transplant. Its use in the treatment of neurological disorder is highly experimental and much additional research is needed in order to test the efficacy of the method in any particular disorder. In the United Stated the Office of Technological Assessment, the analytical arm of the US Congress, is responsible for overseeing this type of research. Best known in this respect is the treatment of Parkinson's disease.

There was a lucky breakthrough by serendipity in the treatment of this condition. The discovery of methyl-phenyl-tetrahydropyridine (MPTP), due to inaccurate synthesis of heroin by an amateur chemist, allowed the first satisfactory animal model for the disorder to be obtained and proved a major advance in itself. It, for the first time, produced an animal model on which different materials could be tested as chronic implants. A variety of tissues have been tried but fetal central nervous material appears to be the most effective in producing dopamine in the brain, the substance deficient in parkinsonism. This raises, apart from any other considerations, the question of ethics, which is complicated.

Bearing in mind that Parkinson's disease is one of the commoner chronic neurological disorders, the limited use of neural grafting can be appreciated by the fact that by 1990 only 3000–4000 patients worldwide had received such treatment. It was an area of initial enthusiasm but clearly one in which very detailed further research needs to be undertaken. Basic animal experimentation is the key to the likelihood of succeeding with the individual patient.

There are other contenders for neural grafts. Alzheimer's disease, Huntington's chorea, and motorneuron disease seem to be strong candidates, but epilepsy is worth detailed consideration. As in parkinsonism so for epilepsy, the disorder and the treatment surround one basic neurotransmitter, in the case of epilepsy, GABA. Neural grafts which could provide additional GABA targeted to the particular area that shows an active spike discharge, could conceivably be more effective than the 'blunderbuss' approach of hoping to block gamma destructive pathways throughout the nervous system (see Chapter 11). This is still all in the future.

PSYCHOLOGICAL TREATMENT

So far this book has been mainly concerned with the drug treatment of epilepsy. I do not, however, underestimate psychosocial factors but these have been reviewed in many texts.

Here it is proposed briefly to refer to behavioural approaches to treatment. These have recently been outlined by Goldstein[8]. There are many interesting leads, even considering methodological difficulties. Some techniques take into account the EEG seizure discharge and use a biofeedback technique to allow the patient to be aware of the discharge, to control it and block the occurrence of the actual clinical attack. The fact that the patients play an active part often appeals to them, rather than the continuous round of tablet-taking, although a combination of the two techniques may be necessary. One can not, however, deny the strong placebo element intrinsic in the use of the complex, if miniaturized, electronic biofeedback apparatus which is needed.

Another procedure using alpha biofeedback can be effective. The alpha rhythm in the EEG can be considered functionally as indicating relaxation. Confirming this is the clinical observation of its absence in the anxious individual. Encouragement of the rhythm, which is fed back electronically to the patient as sound or light, can add to relaxation and is effective[9].

Stress is one of the factors leading to increase in seizures, though not the trigger for the attack itself. Nevertheless, achieving relaxation either by psychotherapeutic approaches or the strategies of the cognitive psychological method may be effective. The patients initially can construct for themselves a detailed list of seizures and any relationship to stressful situations whether it is school, work or in the home. Then specific strategies can be applicable at the stressful points to change lifestyle with benefit.

ALTERNATIVE THERAPY

Many patients with continuing seizures, in spite of adequate medication, frequently ask about alternative means of treatment. The approaches outlined above could possibly be appropriate here. Consideration of newer surgical techniques in patients where conventional methods are not available could also be helpful when the patient feels that the situation is unchanged (see below). Some are able to tolerate the fact that their seizures are unlikely to be ameliorated, others, as with chronic disorders like multiple sclerosis, look elsewhere often without reference to their medical advisers.

The growth of complementary therapy in recent years is not only an expression of the failure of treatment in chronic conditions, but also the patient's feeling that the doctor is not totally aware of the impact of the illness on the whole individual, or that there has been failure to communicate adequately. If rapport has been established with the patient, and this is not always possible, difficulties would not arise. How frequently do we hear the statement that, 'I just could not get on with that doctor, therapist, surgeon, etc., now I feel confident about my treatment and the situation is different'. Other patients contact alternative therapists admitting this only later to their physicians.

Possible dangers

In the course of many years experience in the field, several of my patients have subsequently recounted their experiences. They range from visits to religious centres such as Lourdes, to prolonged treatment with acupuncturists, homeopathists, hypnotists or faith healers. Obviously one does not have an accurate follow-up of any of these, or the various herbal remedies that have been tried. My experience is that, perhaps sadly, alternative therapy does not appear to be the answer in chronic epilepsy. Benefits are transient placebo effects of therapists and medication, just as the introduction of new conventional drugs in resistant cases only results in a short-lived 'honeymoon' for some patients.

It is important to emphasize, if possible, two aspects to the patient *before* they consult alternative therapists. First of all, they must not be foolhardy in reducing medication at the instruction of such a therapist. In my experience serious relapses of seizures, including status epilepticus, have occurred if such advice was not heeded. Also of great importance are the financial considerations. Many patients and their families seek experimental and untried therapy in serious diseases. I warn them, concerning this matter, that the cost may outweigh the benefit, and in any case money is important for the carers of those suffering from chronic disorders so they can, for example, purchase a car, or fund modification of life at home.

ADVANCES IN SURGICAL TREATMENT

Epilepsy surgery, whose history was reviewed in Chapter 7, currently shows a considerable revival[10-12]. This is partly because of the introduction of newer investigatory procedures on the EEG side, coupled with telemetry and split-screen video presentation, of the patient and the EEG simultaneously. Magnetic stimulation methods as well as investigation by magnetic resonance imaging have also been helpful. Such techniques allow refinement of surgical procedures so that operations such as amygdala–hippocampectomy, devised by Yasargil and colleagues[13], may be performed. Results from these procedures are promising, giving intractable patients new hope, and have caused great interest in the UK for a major new impetus to fund surgical centres where research into treatment methods can be carried out. Previous approaches, such as the use of chronic cerebellar stimulation and corpus callosal section, although they seemed interesting advances at the time, have proved to be largely a forlorn hope.

PREVENTION

No book on epilepsy can be complete without attention, at least in passing, to possible preventative means and we may well be at the beginning of a new era in this respect, through the recently developed field of molecular genetics.

The new genetics includes all aspects of the ability to manipulate DNA *in vitro*. It has been an area in which the rapidity of progress is explained by the current concentration of scientific manpower. It reflects the potential importance to basic biological questions, that require answers speedily, not least because there is a change in the demography of the population in developed countries where there is a very marked increase in the older age groups. Coupled with this is the failure of therapeutic breakthroughs in treatment of chronic inherited disorders. There have, therefore, been rapid moves from the laboratory, to applications in practice and indeed no medical specialty has been spared from the potential of such advances.

Taking one particular example, Duchenne muscular dystrophy, the disorder has been investigated in detail and there is now a possibility of direct detection of molecular pathology in prenatal screening. This is not one isolated condition – there are possibilities for the study of other disorders such as cystic fibrosis, neurofibromatosis, haemophilia and Huntington's disease, which might yield to the newer medical genetic techniques, where previously carrier detection and prenatal diagnosis have been unreliable.

There are much broader implications, in that treatment could also be developed directly after detailed determination of abnormal chromosome patterns.

Clinical molecular genetics is also applicable to microbiology where not only are diagnostic procedures important, but they lead directly to therapeutic agents. Such approaches can be developed by study of cell cultures, a technique which is relatively inexpensive and much less time-consuming than many animal-based investigations. Indeed it has been predicted that molecular genetics will occupy a central role in medicine as it moves firmly in the 1990s towards a new century.

GENETIC ASPECTS OF EPILEPSY

It has long been known that there is an inherited element to epilepsy especially in patients with generalized rather than focal seizures, but, in particular, those with a myoclonic disorder (see below). Renewed interest in this aspect has recently come about because of these newer molecular genetic techniques. Until there was this advance most geneticists thought epilepsy was not only too common but almost too complex to justify study in detail[14]. There was also the inaccessibility of the brain preventing direct studies on tissues, which might have reflected on genetic difference susceptibility. In addition population and family studies have not given consistent data about risks. Newer strategies for visualization of the brain allowed a clearer description of individual variations in underlying pathology. However, much more important were the studies at cellular and molecular levels. Genes can now be cloned, matched and sequenced. Although it will be some time before the genetic approaches yield information, already there are some pointers to the fact that unravelling the genetics is possible.

Twin studies and detailed family trees of several generations can yield useful information, but the diagnosis of a particular type of epilepsy can be difficult. Clearly discrete syndromes are of great importance in any detailed study. One group so far investigated is those patients with juvenile myoclonic epilepsy syndrome[15]. Here, not only did the clinical aspect of epilepsy need to be taken into consideration, but also abnormal EEG patterns. When gene mapping was carried out on the basis of the clinical syndrome, there was no evidence of any specific molecular genetic results. However, when this was combined with the EEG findings there was strong evidence for linkage; this was then found to be on chromosome 6.

Febrile convulsions

Another group studied have been those who suffer from febrile convulsions. There is a strong effect of family history in this condition. If parents had had febrile convulsions almost 40% of the siblings will be affected. This suggests that an autosomal dominant pattern would be an appropriate hypothesis. It is known in genetic studies on

Table 3 Antiepileptic compounds at various stages of clinical development in the early 1990s (alphabetically, not in order of possible significance)

Clobazam	Progabide
Denzimol	Oxcarbazepine
Eterobarb	Ralitoline
Felbamate	Stiripentol
Flunarazine	Topiramate
Gabapentin	Vigabatrin
Lamotrigine	Zonisamide
Milacemide	

insects, such as *Drosophila*, that temperature sensitive mutations occur which involve sodium and potassium ion channels[16]. This is a particularly important observation since it is known that phenytoin, for example, has a direct effect on ion channels, and so may furnish a genetic link not only in terms of the epilepsy itself, but also on which antiepileptic drugs may be effective in a particular patient. Further work on finding DNA markers is clearly appropriate. Already, indeed, using DNA probes, a sodium channel gene has been mapped to chromosome 2.

There are obviously great research opportunities in this field. They clearly require careful attention to classification of seizures, delineation of particular syndromes and study of multi-generation families. Obviously the best results will come from collaborative work between clinicians, geneticists and other scientists.

CONCLUSION

It is only 150 years since the effective medical treatment of epilepsy began. Considerable progress has been made and there are currently about 15 substances (see Table 3) at various stages of testing – compounds discovered by detailed screening, perhaps the most important single factor and therapeutic advance[17]. Whether this list contains the miracle drug remains to be seen. The molecular genetic approach suggests that it may offer hope in this direction. Some of the other areas mentioned in this chapter furnish possibilities for the future[18]. It would appear that we must be expectant rather than ecstatic about the possibility of a major breakthrough by the end of the 1990s.

REFERENCES

1. Cereghino, J.J. and Penry, J.K. (1972). Testing of anticonvulsants in man. In Woodbury, D.M., Penry, J.K. and Schmidt, R.P. (eds.) *Anti-epileptic drugs*, 1st edn., (New York: Raven Press)
2. Mann, R.D. (1991). Regulatory Affairs. In Balentyne, B., Marrs, T. and Turner, P.M. *Textbook of General and Applied Regulatory Affairs.* (London: Macmillan)
3. Bishop, J.M. (1990). The Nobel Prize Annual, 1989. (New York: IMG Publishing)
4. Sullivan, J. (1991). Tackling disease with soil and serendipity. *Hospital Doctor*, 30th May
5. Putnam, T.J. and Merritt, H.H. (1937). Experimental determination of the anticonvulsant properties of some phenyl derivatives. *Science*, **85**, 525
6. Marsh, P. (1989). Prescribing all the the way to the bank. *New Scientist*, 18th November
7. Grattini, S. (1991). Need for change in patents for drugs. *Lancet*, **333**, 494
8. Goldstein, H. (1990). Behavioural and cognitive-behavioural treatment for epilepsy: a progress review. *Br. J. Clin. Psychol.*, **29**, 257
9. Cabral, R.J. and Scott, D.F. (1976). Effect of two desensitization techniques, biofeedback and relaxation, on intractable epilepsy: Follow up study. *J. Neurol. Neurosurg. Psychiatr.*, **39**, 504
10. Engel, J.J. (ed.) (1987). *Surgical Treatment of Epilepsies.* (New York: Raven Press)
11. Wieser, H.G. and Elger, C.E. (eds.) (1987). *Presurgical Evaluation of Epileptics.* (Berlin: Springer-Verlag)
12. Editorial. (1988). Surgery for temporal lobe epilepsy. *Lancet*, **2**, 1115
13. Yasargil, M.G., Teddy, P.J. *et al.* (1985). Selective amygdalo-hippocampectomy. Operative anatomy and surgical technique. In Symon, L. (ed.) *Advances and Technical Standards in Neurosurgery*, **12**, 93 (Vienna: Springer-Verlag)
14. Anderson, V.E., Hansen, W.A. and Peary, J.K. (1982). *The Genetic Basis of Epilepsy.* (New York: Raven Press)
15. Meierkord, H. (1989). Advances in genetics and their application to epilepsy. In Trimble, M.R. (ed.) *Chronic Epilepsy, its Prognosis and Management.* (Chichester, UK: Wiley)
16. Salkoff, L.B. and Tanouye, M.A. (1986). Genetics of ion channels. *Physiol. Rev.*, **66**, 301
17. Maxwell, R.A. and Eckhardt, S.B. (1990). *Drug Discovery: A Casebook and Analysis.* (New Jersey: Hamora Press)
18. Leppik, I.E. (1991). Epilepsy: diagnostic and treatment strategies for the next decade. *Epilepsia*, **32**, (Suppl. 5)

Index